Inclusive Child Development Accounts

T0260197

Inclusive Child Development Accounts showcases the global context of emerging asset-building policies and programs around Child Development Accounts.

Child Development Accounts (CDAs) are subsidized accounts that enable families to accumulate assets to invest in children's development and life goals, such as postsecondary education, homeownership, business development, and retirement security. The vision for CDAs is to be universal (meaning everyone participates), progressive (meaning greater subsidies for the poor), and lifelong (meaning from the cradle to the grave). Since 1991, schools, communities, states, provinces, and entire countries have launched various CDA programs and policies. In the first part of the volume, scholars highlight the core feature of "inclusiveness" of CDAs in Singapore, Israel, and the United States. In the second part, scholars report on CDA policies and projects in Taiwan, Uganda, Korea, and mainland China.

Showing how asset building can be effective in diverse cultural and social contexts, and that all these contexts emphasize the investing in children early in life and empowering of them to achieve their potential as productive citizens, *Inclusive Child Development Accounts* will be of great interest to scholars of social work, policy, investment, and development, as well as financial inclusivity. It was originally published as a special issue of the *Asia Pacific Journal of Social Work and Development*.

Jin Huang is Associate Professor in Social Work at the College for Public Health and Social Justice, St. Louis University, USA.

Li Zou is International Director at the Next Age Institute and Center for Social Development, Washington University in St. Louis, USA.

Michael Sherraden is the George Warren Brown Distinguished University Professor and Founding Director at the Center for Social Development, Washington University in St. Louis, USA.

Inclusive Child Development Accounts

Toward Universality and Progressivity

Edited by
Jin Huang, Li Zou and Michael Sherraden

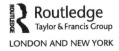

Routledge
Taylor & Francis Group

LONDON AND NEW YORK

First published in paperback 2024

First published 2020
by Routledge
4 Park Square, Milton Park, Abingdon, Oxon OX14 4RN

and by Routledge
605 Third Avenue, New York, NY 10158

Routledge is an imprint of the Taylor & Francis Group, an informa business

Publisher's Note
The publisher has gone to great lengths to ensure the quality of this reprint but points out that some imperfections in the original copies may be apparent.

Disclaimer
Every effort has been made to contact copyright holders for their permission to reprint material in this book. The publishers would be grateful to hear from any copyright holder who is not here acknowledged and will undertake to rectify any errors or omissions in future editions of this book.

British Library Cataloguing-in-Publication Data
A catalogue record for this book is available from the British Library

ISBN: 978-0-367-36979-8 (hbk)
ISBN: 978-1-03-283890-8 (pbk)
ISBN: 978-0-429-35444-1 (ebk)

DOI: 10.4324/9780429354441

Typeset in Minion Pro
by Apex CoVantage, LLC

Contents

CONTENTS

Citation Information

The chapters in this book were originally published in the *Asia Pacific Journal of Social Work and Development*, volume 29, issue 1 (2019). When citing this material, please use the original page numbering for each article, as follows:

Part II Chapter 1

Part II Chapter 2

Part II Chapter 3

Part II Chapter 4

For any permission-related enquiries please visit:
www.tandfonline.com/page/help/permissions

Notes on Contributors

William Byansi is a social work doctoral student at Washington University in St. Louis, USA. His research interest is in child and adolescent behavioral health services and community development.

Li-Chen Cheng is Professor at the Department of Social Work at National Taiwan University. She is an expert on testing Child Development Accounts and antipoverty measures in Taiwan and advising government officials.

Margaret Clancy is the Policy Director and the Director of College Savings Initiative and SEED for Oklahoma Kids, Center for Social Development, Washington University in St. Louis, USA.

Christopher Damulira is a Data Manager at the ICHAD Center in Uganda. He is interested in public health and child welfare issues.

Suo Deng is Associate Professor at the Sociology Department of Peking University, China. His research focuses on poverty and social policy, particularly in the area of asset building and child welfare policies. Dr. Deng currently serves as Deputy Director of Peking University-Hong Kong Polytechnic University China Social Work Research Centre.

Daniel Gottlieb, PhD, is the Deputy Director General of Research and Planning at the National Insurance Institute of Israel, and Associate Professor on Economic Policy and Social Policy at the School of Social Work in the Hebrew University of Jerusalem. His research focuses on social economic policy, in particular on the issues of poverty and the labor market. Over the years he has published many research studies in professional journals, and has written chapters in books on economy and society.

Michal Grinstein-Weiss, PhD, is the Shanti K. Khinduka Distinguished Professor and Associate Dean for Policy Initiatives at the Brown School at Washington University in St. Louis, USA. She serves as director of the university-wide Social Policy Institute at Washington University in St. Louis and as a Nonresident Senior Fellow at the Brookings Institution.

Chang-Keun Han is an expert on development and evaluation of asset-based policy.

Jin Huang is Associate Professor at School of Social Work, St. Louis University, USA, and a faculty director of inclusion in asset building at Center for Social Development, Washington University in St. Louis.

Apollo Kivumbi is the in-country Principal Investigator for SMART Africa-Uganda. He is interested in child and adolescent mental health intervention research.

Olga Kondratjeva, PhD, is the Postdoctoral Research Associate at the Social Policy Institute at Washington University in St. Louis, USA. Her research interests include financial inclusion, financial capability, and the issues of economic and social well-being in the context of the United States and internationally.

Vernon Loke, PhD, is Associate Dean of the College of Social Sciences and Professor of Social Work at Eastern Washington University, USA. He is also a Faculty Associate at the Center for Social Development, Washington University in St Louis. His scholarly interests include asset building and economic empowerment of disadvantaged populations, and the advancement of financial capability in social work.

Miriam Mukasa is Head of Operations at the ICHAD Center in Uganda. She is interested in organizational psychology and worker motivation issues.

Proscovia Nabunya is Research Assistant Professor at Washington University in St. Louis, USA. Her research is focused on social support systems, HIV/AIDS, and poverty-reduction strategies for children and families affected by HIV/AIDS.

Yunju Nam is Associate Professor at the School of Social Work, University at Buffalo, State University of New York, USA.

Phionah Namatovu is Project Coordinator for ICHAD and SMART Africa-Uganda. She is interested in evidence-based practices to improve child behavioral health outcomes.

Jennifer Nattabi, MSW, is a Research Coordinator at the International Center for Child Health and Development at Washington University in St. Louis. She is interested in girl child empowerment and child welfare issues.

Ofir Pinto, PhD, is Director of the Planning Policy Unit in the Research and Planning Department at the National Insurance Institute of Israel. He is interested in applying insights from economics and psychology in the context of social problems and public policy.

Stephen P. Roll, PhD, is Research Assistant Professor at the Brown School at Washington University in St. Louis, USA. His research focuses on promoting asset building, debt management, and financial stability in financially vulnerable populations.

Michael Sherraden is the George Warren Brown Distinguished University Professor and Founding Director, Center for Social Development and Next Age Institute, Washington University in St. Louis, USA.

Fred M. Ssewamala is Professor at Washington University in St. Louis, USA. His research is focused on innovative economic empowerment and social protection interventions for children and youth in sub-Saharan Africa.

Li Zou is the International Director, Center for Social Development and Next Age Institute, Washington University in St. Louis, USA.

Foreword

This book exemplifies the focused, purposeful nature of Child Development Account (CDA) policies and programs as social innovation. Given the global perspectives illuminated in the chapters of this book, a clearer picture emerges that CDAs did not simply arise—they were deliberately and rigorously conceived, proposed, implemented, and tested. In each country's CDA discussed herein, the policy features, circumstances, and cultural considerations differ in important ways. Despite such differences, the long-term vision of the CDAs across the globe remains consistent: to support the growth and development of all children to ensure their greatest potential.

We believe this represents a small example of the best humans have to offer. As a highly social species, our "best thing" has been to shape social arrangements and institutions to make the world a better place. Indeed, human sociality and innovation make all other aspects of human development possible. Humans do not always get social innovation right—history is littered with mistaken social organization of one kind or another. In the case of CDAs, however, the evidence consistently confirms that such policy can be implemented and sustained to deliver positive outcomes.

It is not a coincidence that CDAs as a social innovation are emerging during a global period of increased financialization and rising inequality. As the world rapidly becomes increasingly financialized, the people without financial capability are pushed farther and farther to the margins. Exacerbating this trend is the staggering pace at which global wealth is rising to the top. Because assets are necessary for *all people* to invest in their growth and development, this inequality is not only a moral failing, but also a huge loss of human potential. Designed in the context of these circumstances, CDAs promote inclusive financial capability and wealth accumulation for all.

The CDA innovation is emerging—seeds are sprouting—but CDA policy has not yet spread widely and grown into a stable social innovation everywhere. There is a long way to go, but we have made encouraging progress. In the process, scholars and policymakers are learning a great deal from each other, and the growing body of evidence continuously informs and improves CDA policies as more countries adopt and implement them.

For example, since the December 2017 CDA symposium (which this book covers), universal CDA policies have emerged in several U.S. states, including California, Illinois, and Nebraska (all in 2019) and Pennsylvania (2018). These states join Maine, Rhode Island, Connecticut, and Nevada, which enacted statewide CDA policies in earlier years.

The Taiwan government is now working to change their existing CDA program from an "opt-in" policy to "opt-out" policy, based on research evidence on CDAs in the United

States. This policy change could potentially increase the CDA participation rate from 45% of all eligible Taiwanese children to almost 100%.

Though difficult to predict the shifting economic and policy landscapes in the years ahead, it seems likely that most countries will continue to face rising financialization, widening asset inequity, high costs of higher education, and a necessity to prepare each new generation for highly skilled labor and engaged citizenship. In these circumstances, CDAs can contribute positively by providing every child with sound financial footing and promoting economic and social development for society overall.

We are grateful to Routledge/Taylor & Francis for selecting our special journal issue to be developed into this book. We have appreciated working with Lydia de Cruz, the Commissioning Editor at Taylor & Francis. We thank Lee Geok Ling of National University of Singapore and Amy Quon of Routledge/Taylor & Francis for their kind assistance in the book preparation, and John Gabbert of Washington University in St. Louis for his always thorough editorial work for both the special journal issue and this book.

Michael Sherraden

Jin Huang

Li Zou

St. Louis, October 2019

Toward universal, progressive, and lifelong asset building: introduction to the special issue on inclusive child development accounts

Michael Sherraden, Jin Huang and Li Zou

ABSTRACT

Child Development Accounts (CDAs) are subsidised savings or investment accounts that enable families to accumulate assets to invest in
children's long-term development. Ideally, CDAs are universal (everyone participates), progressive (greater subsidies for the poor) and lifelong (beginning at birth). This introduction provides a theoretical and
policy background of CDAs in the global context, summarises seven
papers in this volume and creates a vision for future CDA development.

Child Development Accounts (CDAs) are subsidised savings or investment accounts that enable families to accumulate assets to invest in children's development and life course goals, such as postsecondary education, home purchase, small business development and retirement security. CDAs are envisioned as universal (everyone participates), progressive (greater subsidies for the poor) and potentially lifelong (beginning at birth) national policy (Sherraden, 1991, 2014). Since the concept was proposed (Sherraden, 1991), many CDA programmes and policies have been created at different levels, ranging across schools, communities, cities, states/provinces and countries, with varied designs and operations.

To aid the transition from the industrial era into a globalised, information-era economy, social policies must go beyond supporting consumption: they must create opportunities for individuals to invest in long-term development. Thus, many countries are exploring new policy innovations that encourage asset building, including CDAs. This special issue aims to present the latest policy developments and research findings on CDAs in a global context, including examples in the Asia-Pacific region.

Background

Assets, as the stock of economic resources, enable people to make investments that expand their capabilities and improve their long-term circumstances – for example, investments in education, homes or enterprise. Assets also enable people to finance irregular expenses, purchase large-ticket items and weather financial crises (Paxton, 2001, 2002; Sherraden, 1991). Asset-based policy complements income-based policy to promote family economic well-being. However, existing asset-based policies are often regressive, supporting the well-off through tax benefits (Howard, 1997; Sherraden, 1991; Woo, Rademacher, & Meier, 2010). In contrast, the CDAs discussed in this special issue are designed to achieve inclusive asset building for all, especially low-income and financially vulnerable families.

Ideally, CDAs are universal, progressive and lifelong (Sherraden, 1991, 2014). To include everyone, they should be automatically opened for all newborns with initial deposits. Research consistently shows that voluntary (non-automatic) asset-building programmes will both fail to be universal, and also exclude economically disadvantaged families (Congressional Budget Office, 2011; Dynarski, 2004; Government Accountability Office, 2012; Springstead & Wilson, 2000; U.S.). CDAs can offer progressive subsidies for economically disadvantaged families, such as larger initial deposits, additional deposits over time and greater savings' matches. Recent research suggests key design elements to achieve these goals (Clancy & Beverly, 2017).

Asset accumulation is a long-term process. Starting CDAs early in life (ideally at birth) allows more time to generate investment earnings (Beverly, Clancy, Huang, & Sherraden, 2015). Lifelong CDAs can support a variety of life course investments: education and experiences in early childhood, success in post-secondary education adulthood, and homeownership and retirement stability in later life. Having a single account that follows an individual from birth to retirement is the most efficient way to make asset policy lifelong.

In addition to financial benefits, CDAs have positive effects on attitudes and behaviours of parents and children, such as educational expectations, parenting practice, maternal depression and social–emotional development (e.g. Elliott, Choi, Destin, & Kim, 2011; Grinstein-Weiss, Williams Shanks, & Beverly, 2014; Williams Shanks, Kim, Loke, & Destin, 2010).

CDA papers in this volume

This special issue builds upon the December 2017 *International Symposium on Inclusion in Asset Building: Policy Innovation and Social Impacts* at the National University of Singapore. The symposium was organised by the Next Age Institute, a partnership on social innovation between Washington University in St. Louis and the National University of Singapore. We have organised this special issue in two broad parts: (1) inclusive CDA policies, and (2) CDA programmes and projects.

The three articles in Part 1 highlight the core feature of 'inclusiveness' of CDAs in Singapore, Israel and the United States. In the first, Vernon Loke and Michael Sherraden analyse Singapore's comprehensive asset-based social policies, with four national programmes building assets for all children – the Baby Bonus and CDAs, Edusave Accounts, Post-Secondary Education Accounts (PSEAs) and Medisave Accounts. These four accounts in practice function as an integrated CDA policy that is linked to the accountholder's Central Provident Fund as an adult. The second article by Michal Grinstein-Weiss, Olga Kondratjeva, Stephen P. Roll, Ofir Pinto and Daniel Gottlieb provides an overview of the Israel's newly implemented universal CDA programme, the Saving for Every Child Programme, and details its implementation and early findings. In the third article, Jin Huang, Yunju Nam, Michael Sherraden and Margaret Clancy report that a universal CDA experiment in the US state of Oklahoma, known as SEED OK, significantly reduces punitive-parenting behaviours among treatment mothers with young children. This finding joins other SEED OK studies that document positive attitudinal and behaviour changes generated from CDAs (Sherraden et al., 2015).

Part 2 covers CDA programmes and projects in four countries. Li-Chen Cheng investigates Taiwan's Children Future Education and Development Accounts, describing its core components and future challenges. Proscovia Nabunya, Phionah Namatovu, Christopher Damulira, Apollo Kivumbi, William Byansi, Miriam Mukasa, Jennifer Nattabi, and Fred M. Ssewamala report experimental findings from an asset-building intervention for orphaned and vulnerable children in Uganda, and find that treatment children with CDAs had better academic performance and more successful school transitions.Chang-Keun Han examines Korea's CDAs for institutionalised children, and suggests that CDAs have positive influences on children's mindsets, saving habits, education and future planning. Suo Deng assesses two pilot CDA programmes in Shan'xi province of China. In addition to financial benefits, the pilot CDA programmes improve parent–child interactions and parents' future orientation.

Contributions and directions

These seven papers indicate broad interest in CDAs among policymakers and researchers. They represent the latest CDA policy developments in the global context, adding to the CDA experiences and accomplishments achieved in other countries (e.g. the United Kingdom, Canada). As experience and knowledge continue to build, other countries are also exploring CDA policy options.

Three policies/programmes included in this special issue have adopted automatic enrolment to achieve universal participation for asset building, and all provide financial incentives to disadvantaged families. The CDA examples discussed in this issue start at different stages of childhood and target varied populations. The studies examine a variety of important topics related to CDA policy, including the political context, legislative process, policy design and implementation, and financial and nonfinancial benefits for children and parents. To some extent, these seven policies/programmes also illustrate different policy development stages, such as pilot programmes, demonstration research, policy for special populations, and inclusive asset building for all. Findings of these studies build upon previous evidence from CDA research, and provide research 'triangulation' in different cultural and societal contexts.

In addition to the importance of universality and progressivity, several other lessons generated from these studies may facilitate CDA policy development, promote inclusive asset building and enable all individuals to invest in long-term development. For example, it may be efficient to build CDAs on existing policy vehicles and systems. The SEED OK experiment in the United States is based on a state 529 college savings plan for children, whereas Israel's CDA has a close connection with the Child Allowance programme. The development of newer asset-building policies for children in Singapore is integrated with its overall asset-building strategy as core social policy.

Experiences from all of these studies suggest that asset building can be effective in diverse cultural and social contexts. However, CDA design and implementation must also address specific challenges and goals within each country. This may be reducing child poverty and economic inequality in Taiwan and Israel, targeted poverty alleviation in Mainland China, self-sufficiency of institutionalised children in Korea or support for AIDS orphans in Uganda.

CDA design and implementation may benefit from its integration with new technology. For example, WeChat, a popular social media in China, has been used in the pilot CDA programmes to support parental education. Recently, the implementation of the Baby Bonus in Singapore has been included in its Smart Nation platform. Innovations in financial technology ('fintech') will increasingly be relevant to – and integrated with – social policies. CDAs can help to chart this integration.

The emergence and growth of CDAs around the globe have prompted scholars, policy-makers, government officials and community stakeholders to exchange experiences and lessons, identify global trends and chart future directions. This special issue illuminates CDA innovations in a global context. A longer and more ambitious (yet possible) vision is that innovations in CDAs may lead someday to an asset-building account for every child on the planet. We can imagine a world in which every newborn begins her life with a legal identify (birth registration), a health check-up, necessary immunisations and a CDA to help build her future. The CDA would be a fully inclusive social policy that avoids funding 'leakage', bypasses corruption and connects capital flows directly to secure accounts of individual children all over the world. Consider, for example, international aid that goes directly into children's accounts. The core practice of 'development work' would shift from experts meeting in hotels to money building in accounts of children everywhere. Technically, this vision is already within reach – every child can have a birth registration and an account. To be sure, there are political and institutional barriers of all kinds, but our goal as social policy scholars is to imagine, test, inform and create positive social and economic change. In this pursuit, there is little advantage in thinking small. We would like to think of this set of CDA papers as a useful step along this pathway.

Disclosure statement

We thank colleagues at the National University of Singapore (NUS) for hosting the Child Development Account conference, Lee Geok Ling at NUS for editorial leadership of *Asian Pacific Journal of Social Work and Development*, John Gabbert of Washington University in St. Louis (WU) for editorial work for special issue, and our academic colleagues around the world who have authored this set of papers. No potential conflict of interest was reported by the authors.

References

Beverly, S. G., Clancy, M. M., Huang, J., & Sherraden, M. (2015). *The SEED for Oklahoma Kids child development account experiment: Accounts, assets, earnings, and savings* (CSD Research Brief No. 15–29). St. Louis, MO: Washington University, Center for Social Development.

Clancy, M. M., & Beverly, S. G. (2017). *Statewide child development account policies: Key design elements* (CSD Policy Report No. 17–30). St. Louis, MO: Washington University, Center for Social Development. doi:10.7936/K7G44PS2

Congressional Budget Office. (2011). *Use of tax incentives for retirement saving in 2006.* Washington, DC: Author.

Dynarski, S. (2004). Who benefits from the education saving incentives? Income, educational expectations and the value of the 529 and Coverdell. *National Tax Journal, 57*(2), 359–383.

Elliott, W., III, Choi, E. H., Destin, M., & Kim, K. H. (2011). The age old question, which comes first? A simultaneous test of children's savings and children's college-bound identity. *Children and Youth Services Review, 33*(7), 1101–1111.

Government Accountability Office. (2012). *Higher education: A small percentage of families save in 529 plans* (Report No. GAO-13-64). Washington, DC: Author.

Grinstein-Weiss, M., Williams Shanks, T. R., & Beverly, S. G. (2014). Family assets and child outcomes: Evidence and directions. *The Future of Children, 24*(1), 147–170.

Howard, C. (1997). *The hidden welfare state: Tax expenditures and social policy in the United States.* Princeton, NJ: Princeton University Press.

Paxton, W. (2001). The asset-effect: An overview. In J. Bynner & W. Paxton (Eds.), *The asset-effect* (pp. 1–16). London: Institute for Public Policy Research.

Paxton, W. (2002). Assets and the definition of poverty. In C. Kober & W. Paxton (Eds.), *Asset-based welfare and poverty: Exploring the case for and against asset-based welfare policies* (pp. 9–12). London: National Children's Bureau.

Sherraden, M. (1991). *Assets and the poor: A new American welfare policy.* Armonk, NY: M. E. Sharpe.

Sherraden, M. (2014). Asset building research and policy: Pathways, progress, and potential of a social innovation. In R. Cramer & T. R. Williams Shanks (Eds.), *The assets perspective: The rise of asset building and its impact on social policy* (pp. 263–284). New York: Palgrave Macmillan.

Sherraden, M., Clancy, M., Nam, Y., Huang, J., Kim, Y., Beverly, S. G., ... Purnell, J. Q. (2015). Universal accounts at birth: Building knowledge to inform policy. *Journal of the Society for Social Work and Research, 6*(4), 541–564.

Springstead, G. R., & Wilson, T. M. (2000). Participation in voluntary individual savings accounts: An analysis of IRAs, 401(k)s, and the TSP. *Social Security Bulletin, 63*(1), 34–39.

Williams Shanks, T. R., Kim, Y., Loke, V., & Destin, M. (2010). Assets and child well-being in developed countries. *Children and Youth Services Review, 32*(11), 1488–1496.

Woo, B., Rademacher, I., & Meier, J. (2010). *Upside down: The $400 billion federal asset-building budget.* Washington, DC: Corporation for Enterprise Development and Annie E. Casey Foundation.

Building assets from birth: Singapore's policies

Vernon Loke and Michael Sherraden

ABSTRACT
Singapore has created innovative, inclusive and comprehensive asset-building policies designed to promote social stability and development. Asset building from early childhood is an important part of this overall strategy. In 1993, Singapore's government initiated a universal child asset-building policy, Edusave, which provides resources for improving educational outcomes. Since then, three additional asset-building policies for children have been implemented: the Baby Bonus and Child Development Accounts (CDAs), Post-Secondary Education Accounts (PSEAs) and Medisave, a health savings account. We discuss each of these asset-building accounts for children in Singapore. We point out distinctive features and assess key elements in overall policy design.

Introduction

Singapore has a comprehensive and integrated policy framework for building assets across the life course. Indeed, this is the most prominent theme in Singapore's social policy (Sherraden, 2018). The purposes of this policy theme are to create a nation of asset holders, develop every citizen to reach his or her potential, and promote social stability and development. In this context, four types of asset-building accounts in Singapore focus specifically on children: (1) the Baby Bonus and Child Development Account, (2) Edusave, (3) Post-Secondary Education Accounts, and (4) Medisave for Newborns. These four policies enable children to accumulate assets, and as such, could be categorised together as comprehensive Child Development Accounts (CDAs).

CDAs are subsidised savings or investment accounts that enable children to accumulate assets for life course needs and their social and economic development. Ideally, CDAs are universal, progressive and lifelong, starting at or near birth (Sherraden, 1991; Sherraden, Cheng et al., 2018). In this paper, we review existing research, government data and other publications to present an overview of the asset-building policies that target children in Singapore. We begin by reviewing Singapore's four asset-building accounts that focus on children, assess the design elements of those policies, reflect on their basic features, and conclude with some policy recommendations for other countries seeking to implement similar policies.

Table 1. Baby bonus benefits.

Baby bonus component	Benefits for 1st or 2nd child	Benefits for 3rd or 4th child	Benefits for 5th child onwards
Cash Gift (into parents designated bank account)	S$8,000	S$10,000	S$10,000
First Step Grant (CDA account)	S$3,000	S$3,000	S$3,000
Dollar-for-dollar savings match (CDA account)	Up to S$3,000	Up to S$9,000	Up to S$15,000
Total benefits	Up to S$14,000	Up to S$22,000	Up to S$28,000

Table 2. Ten key CDA policy design elements.

	Edusave Account	Child Development Account (CDA)	Post-Secondary Education Account (PSEA)	Medisave Account and Medisave Grant for Newborns
1. Universal eligibility	Yes	Yes	Yes	Yes
2. Automatic opt-out enrolment	Yes	No	Yes	Yes
3. Automatic initial deposit	Yes	Yes	Yes	Yes
4. Automatic progressive subsidy	No	No	No	No
5. At-birth start	No	Yes	Yes, when integrated with CDA	Yes
6. Centralised savings plan	Yes	Yes	Yes	Yes
7. Targeted investment options	No	No	No	No
8. Potential for investment growth	Limited	Limited	Limited	Limited
9. Restricted withdrawals	Yes	Yes	Yes	Yes
10. Public benefit exclusions	Yes	Yes	Yes	Yes

Asset-building accounts focusing on children

This section summarises Singapore's four asset-building accounts for children – Edusave, Baby Bonus and CDAs, Post-Secondary Education Accounts and Medisave for Newborns – that make up its integrated CDA policy. The policies are presented in the order in which they were established. Though the policies function via asset building, the underlying purposes are to develop individuals and families in Singapore. Objectives for each policy are different, including promoting higher birth rates, supporting families, investing in children, and building human capital. In other words, asset building for children is not an end in itself, but rather a means to achieve important social goals.

Edusave

The *Education Endowment Scheme Act of 1993* established in Singapore is one of the earliest known universal child asset-building policies in the world (Curley & Sherraden, 2000; Loke & Sherraden, 2009, Loke & Sherraden, 2015). Also known as the Edusave Scheme or simply Edusave, this policy aims to enhance the quality of education in Singapore, and to increase educational opportunities for all Singaporean children aged 7–16 years (Singapore Ministry of Education, 2017). Edusave is multifaceted, functioning through grants to support educational institutions; merit awards and scholarships to students; the Edusave Pupil Fund; and Edusave accounts. As with several other social policies in Singapore, Edusave itself is based on underlying assets. A S$1 billion Edusave Endowment Fund was established by the government in 1993, and returns from this fund, which has since grown to S$5.5 billion, support all the programmes in the Edusave Scheme. (At this writing, S$100 is equivalent to US$73).

For this paper, the policy component of interest is the Edusave account. When a child turns 7, he or she automatically receives an Edusave account. Annual government contributions and periodic one-off grants fund these accounts. In 2018, students in primary schools (grades 1–6) receive S$200 in annual contributions, and those in secondary schools receive S$240. Accountholders also receive occasional top-offs in the accounts from the government. For example, in 2015, accountholders received an additional S$150 one-off grant from the government. Such contributions and grants are automatically deposited. Starting in 2019, the annual Edusave contributions from the government will be increased to S$230 for primary-level students and S$290 for secondary-level students (Singapore Ministry of Finance, 2018).

The government is the sole funder of Edusave accounts. The accounts are a receptacle into which the government can deposit annual contributions and periodic grants. There is no provision for additional deposits from other persons or entities. Edusave accountholders can use funds accumulated in Edusave accounts to pay for school fees, other school charges, or enrichment programmes. Balances in these accounts earn guaranteed interest of at least 2.5% per annum. When an accountholder turns 17 or leaves secondary school, any unused balance in the Edusave account is transferred to his or her Post-Secondary Education Account (Singapore Ministry of Education, 2017).

Baby bonus and child development accounts

In 2001, Singapore's government enacted the *Child Development Co-Savings Act*, to both incentivise childbirth among Singaporeans, and also to create an environment conducive to raising families. In addition to the provisions of maternity, paternity, shared-parental, infant-care, and childcare leave, the Act also established the Child Development Co-Savings Scheme. Popularly known as the Baby Bonus Scheme and Child Development Accounts (CDA), the Child Development Co-Savings Scheme has benefitted from several enhancements since its inception, including an increase in benefits and extension of benefits to all Singaporean children. Parents sign up (opt-in) for the Scheme by completing a simple online application form as early as 8 weeks prior to the child's estimated delivery date. Taking less than 10 minutes to complete, the application asks for basic demographic information about the family and child, as well as instructions on which banks the parents designate to receive the benefits.

This asset-building policy comprises two tiers. The first tier is an unrestricted cash gift from the government of S$8,000 for the first and second child, and S$10,000 for each subsequent child. The government disburses this cash gift within 3 weeks after the birth of the child, depositing it directly into a designated parent's bank account in five instalments over 18 months.

The second tier consists of the CDA, which begins with the CDA First Step grant. The CDA is a restricted savings account that the government matches dollar-to-dollar. The CDAs open automatically at a commercial bank the parents designate, within 3–5 working days of the child's birth registration or after the completion of the online application form.

To kickstart savings in the CDAs, the government seeds each account with S$3,000 from the CDA First Step grant. Private contributions to CDAs (usually from parents) are matched by the government up to a cap of S$3,000 for first- and second-born children, S$9,000 for the third- and fourth-born children, and S$15,000 for fifth-born and subsequent children (see Table 1). The co-savings match contribution publicly affirms and supports parents as having the primary responsibility of raising their children. Families can contribute to their children's CDAs and enjoy the savings match until December 31 of the year the child turns 12.

In addition to the CDA First Step grant and the savings match from the government, CDAs also receive periodic top-ups from the government. For example, in 2015, children who were 6 years or younger received an additional top-up of S$300 or S$600 into their CDAs, depending on the household's economic status (Singapore Ministry of Finance, 2015).

At this writing, balances in CDAs earn guaranteed interest of around 2% per annum. Monies in these accounts may be used to cover expenses incurred by the accountholder or their siblings, related to childcare, preschool and kindergarten, and special education or early intervention programmes. Accountholders or their siblings may also use CDA funds for medical care, pharmaceuticals, assistive technology, eye care and health insurance. In sum, the CDA resources target education and health, two key components of human capital. Any unused balance in a child's CDA is later transferred to the child's Post-Secondary Education Account when the child turns 13.

Post-secondary education accounts

First announced in 2005 and established in 2008 by revising the *Education Endowment Scheme Act* to become the *Education Endowment and Savings Schemes Act*, Post-Secondary Education Accounts (PSEAs) are a part of the Singapore government's efforts to encourage every Singaporean to build financial resources to pursue and complete post-secondary education. The balances from CDAs and Edusave accounts are automatically transferred to PSEAs when accountholders turn 13 and 17, respectively. Accountholders who have not reached their savings match cap for CDAs can continue to contribute to their PSEAs and receive matching grants from the government until the savings match cap is attained or when the child turns 18, whichever is earlier.

Like CDAs, PSEAs also receive additional government top-ups periodically. There were five top-ups from 2008 to 2015 (Singapore Ministry of Education, n.d.). The most recent was in 2015, wherein accountholders aged 17–20 received either S$250 or S$500 automatically in their PSEAs, with progressive funding depending on household economic status (Singapore Ministry of Finance, 2015).

Funds in the PSEAs earn interests of at least 2.5% per annum and can be used for approved post-secondary educational expenses. Any unused balances are automatically transferred to the accountholder's Central Provident Fund (CPF) account at the age of 30 years. During fiscal year 2016/2017, S$86.7 million was withdrawn by 225,150 account holders for fees and charges at approved educational institutions. As of 31 March 2017, there was a total balance of S$1.5 billion in PSEAs (Singapore Ministry of Education, 2017).

Though not the focus of this paper, it is important here to briefly summarise the Central Provident Fund, commonly known simply as CPF. The backbone of Singapore's asset-building policy, the CPF is a mandatory savings account into which every employed person contributes, with matched contributions from employers. Though primarily meant for retirement security, CPF savings are also used for medical expenses and for a variety of asset-building purposes such as the purchase of homes, investments, insurances and tertiary educational expenses (Loke & Cramer, 2009; Sherraden, Nair, Vasoo, Liang, & Sherraden, 1995; Vasoo & Singh, 2018). Social and economic impacts of the CPF have been extraordinary, creating assets and contributing to social stability for a very large portion of Singapore's population (Vasoo & Singh, 2018). It is relevant in this discussion, because balances from all the child asset-building accounts described in this paper eventually roll over into the CPF, creating an integrated and lifelong asset-building policy.

Medisave for newborns

In 2013, Singapore's government began automatically opening a Medisave account for every Singaporean newborn upon registration of birth. Established under the *Central Provident Fund Act*, Medisave is a national health-savings scheme to enable CPF members save for future medical expenses (Loke & Cramer, 2009; Sherraden et al., 1995). Funds in the Medisave account can defray the cost of healthcare expenses such as vaccinations, hospitalisations and approved outpatient treatments.

In addition to automatically receiving Medisave accounts, each newborn receives the Medisave Grant for Newborns to help ensure that they begin life with enough resources in their Medisave accounts. In 2013 and 2014, the government automatically deposited S $3,000 into each newborn's Medisave account. The grant amount was subsequently increased to S$4,000 for those born on or after 1 January, 2015 (Singapore Government, n.d.). This increased amount is sufficient to pay for the accountholder's Medishield Life premiums from birth through age 21. Medishield Life is a basic health insurance plan, administered by the Central Provident Fund Board, that helps pay for large hospital bills and selected costly outpatient treatment, thereby reducing patient's Medisave and cash outlays for these medical events and needs.

Assessing Singapore's asset-building policies for children: key policy design elements for CDAs

Child Development Accounts are envisioned to be universal, progressive and potentially lifelong (Sherraden, Clancy, et al., 2018). To be the most successful, CDAs should ideally incorporate the following design elements (described in detail by Clancy & Beverly, 2017): (1) universal eligibility; (2) automatic opt-out enrolment; (3) automatic initial deposit; (4) automatic progressive subsidy; (5) at-birth start; (6) centralised savings plan; (7) targeted investment options; (8) potential for investment growth; (9) restricted withdrawals; and (10) exclusion of other public benefits when determining eligibility (see Table 2).

The first four design elements are essential to address economic inequality via full participation and greater public support for those who need it most. Accounts starting at birth, element 5, maximises the time available for contributions to be made into these accounts, for balances to grow over time, and for positive psychological effects of asset ownership to develop. Holding accounts in centralised structures, element 6, creates economies of scale and reduces administrative burden in managing the accounts. With targeted investment options, element 7, that provide potential for growth, element 8, decision-making at account opening is simplified, while simultaneously maximising investment returns that could add substantially to total balances in CDAs over time. Restricting withdrawals, element 9, ensures that CDA funds are used for intended purposes. And finally, exclusion of other public benefits, element 10, ensures that accountholders are not denied or penalised for accumulating assets in the CDAs when applying for any other public assistance. In the following section, we use these 10 CDA design elements to assess the four Singaporean CDA policies.

Universal eligibility

All Singaporean children are now eligible to benefit from the four policies detailed in this paper. However, with the exception of the Medisave grant for newborns, which had universal eligibility at its inception in 2013, the other three programmes were not universal until recently. For Edusave accounts between 1993 and 2014, only students enrolled in schools that were funded by Singapore's Ministry of Education were eligible to have the accounts opened. Singaporean children enrolled in private or religious schools, home-schooled or residing overseas were left out of the Edusave programme. Only in 2014 did eligibility to receive Edusave benefits extend to all Singaporean children aged 7–16.

When the Baby Bonus was first implemented in 2001, eligibility was initially restricted to only the second- and third-birth-order children born within wedlock in each family. In 2004, the government extended eligibility for the Baby Bonus to the first four children in each family born to married parents, with the first-born child receiving the cash gift but not the CDA, whereas the second- to fourth-order children received both the cash gift and CDA benefits (Steering Group on Population, 2004). It further extended eligibility to all children born within wedlock in 2008, with all children receiving both the cash gift as well as CDA benefits (Singapore Prime Minister's Office, 2008). And in 2016, the government announced that children of unwed parents born on or after September 2016 will also be eligible to receive CDA benefits. However, these children will not be eligible to receive the cash gift (Singapore Ministry of Social and Family Development, 2016). Thus, the long-term policy trajectory is towards greater inclusion.

With regard to the PSEAs, as the accounts were initially established to receive rollover balances from CDAs and Edusave accounts, eligibility was limited to the extent that CDAs and Edusave were limited. However, with Edusave being extended to all Singaporean students in 2014, PSEAs now also feature universal eligibility from that point. In addition, PSEAs are automatically opened, if one does not yet exist, to receive the periodic PSEA government top-ups. With the most recent PSEA top-up to all Singaporeans aged 17–20 years in 2015, universality was achieved.

Automatic opt-out enrolment

With the exception of the Baby Bonus, the other three CDA policies reviewed in this paper feature automatic (opt-out) enrolment, with Medisave accounts opened automatically upon birth registration, Edusave accounts opened automatically when the child turns 7, and PSEAs opened automatically when the child turns 13.

Regarding the Baby Bonus, parents are required to opt-in to enrol in the policy, but the application is simple – completion of an online form that takes less than 10 minutes. The online application asks for basic information to establish citizenship of parents, information about birth or impending birth of the child, parents' preferred mode of communication, and designated bank account to receive the cash gift and CDA funds. The CDA is then automatically opened at the bank of choice after the birth of the child. Parents do not have to visit the bank for account opening. Parents can complete the online application as early as 8 weeks before the estimated delivery date of the child, or afterbirth registration. Parents may also receive assistance in completing the application from any of the maternity hospitals, any of the 26 Citizen Connect Centres across the country, or at the point of birth registration.

Automatic initial deposit

Overall, the various CDA policies in Singapore have automatic initial deposit integrated into their designs where appropriate. As previously indicated, the S$4,000 Medisave grant for Newborns are automatically deposited into the child's Medisave account around the time of birth. As for Edusave accounts, the government makes annual deposits automatically. Initial deposits are not applicable to PSEAs, as they are designed to receive unused balances rolled over from CDAs and Edusave.

For the Baby Bonus, the cash gift component is automatically deposited into the designated parent's bank account in five payments over 18 months, with the first payment deposited within 10 days of birth. Parents have the option of redepositing this unrestricted cash gift into their child's CDA if they so wish. As for the CDA, the Singapore government implemented automatic initial deposits for children born on as of March 2016 through the CDA First Step grant. With this enhancement to the CDA, all children have an S$3,000 grant deposited automatically within 2 weeks of account opening.

Automatic progressive subsidy

The CDA policies reviewed in this paper are not envisioned as residual social welfare policy designed to assist the poor and vulnerable. Rather, they are fully inclusive, intended to achieve positive social outcomes for every child in the country, regardless of economic background. The policies do not have progressive subsidies built directly into their designs, but the Singapore government periodically provides additional top-up grants to the PSEAs and CDAs on a progressive basis. The top-up amount is usually tied to household economic status, with lower income households receiving more. funds. For example, in 2015, children from lower income households received an additional S$600 and S$500 in their CDA and PSEA accounts, respectively, whereas those from higher income households received half that amount.

At-birth start

Strictly speaking, only the Medisave and CDA accounts begin at or near birth, whereas the Edusave accounts are opened when the child begins school in the year they turn 7, and the PSEAs are opened in the year the account holder turns 13. However, CDAs, Edusave and PSEAs are integrated with each other, with balances in CDAs and Edusave automatically rolling over into the PSEAs. In this important sense, it would not be inaccurate to interpret Singapore's CDA policy overall as collectively starting at birth.

Centralised savings plan and potential for investment growth

Singapore's CDAs are largely centrally managed, with the Central Provident Fund Board administering Medisave accounts, and Singapore's Ministry of Education administering Edusave and PSEAs. The government initially managed CDAs but subsequently transferred management to a few large commercial banks.

Unlike in the United States, where most CDAs have different investment options, CDA programmes in Singapore are primarily savings products with modest fixed returns. The accounts have been earning interest at 2% to 2.5% in recent years, higher than market rate for most savings products. Though there is no market risk associated with Singaporean CDAs, there is also limited upside potential.

Restricted withdrawals and public benefits exclusions

With the exception of the unrestricted cash gift of the Baby Bonus, savings in the various CDAs are protected and can only be withdrawn for approved purposes of human capital development. For example, accountholders can use funds in Medisave for approved medical expenses or to purchase health insurance, whereas they can use Edusave funds for approved school fees or educational enrichment programmes. Savings in CDAs can be used for expenses related to childcare, early intervention programmes, or for healthcare, whereas funds in PSEAs can be used to help pay for post-secondary education.

As noted, the CDA policies reviewed in this paper are not designed to target the poor and economically disadvantaged. As such, funds accumulated in CDAs are not taken into consideration in the determination of eligibility for any public benefits in Singapore. This approach differs from CDAs in other countries; for example, CDA funds are considered when applying for Temporary Assistance to Needy Families in the United States (Clancy & Beverly, 2017).

Reflections on Singapore's asset-building framework

Singapore represents an interesting case study in asset building. It is one of just a few countries where 'asset enhancement' is the bedrock of social welfare and economic development policies. Though no policy is perfect, Singapore has made strides in promoting asset building for children over the years. In this section, we reflect on the basic features of Singapore's approach to social policy. These features include alignment with societal values, a lifelong framework, universal eligibility and automatic enrolment, substantial government investment, constant evolution and potential for investment growth.

Alignment with, and leveraging upon, societal values and priorities

One reason for Singapore's strong support for asset building is that it aligns with, and leverages upon, the people and government's values and priorities. The government sees its role as a creator of an environment conducive to asset building for all, rather than a provider of income subsidies (Sung, 2006). The CDA policies discussed above are part of this larger endeavour.

Strongly related to this, as a geographically small nation state with no natural resources, Singapore's greatest asset is its people (Tarmugi, 1995). As a result, Singapore values and emphasises human capital development (Haskins, 2011). The various CDA policies reflect human capital development through their focus on education and healthcare.

Short-term targeted accounts embedded in a life-long framework of asset building

Related to the human capital theme, Singapore's asset-building accounts are somewhat short-term in duration, designed to meet specific developmental needs at particular junctures during childhood into the early adulthood. As discussed, funds in Medisave and CDAs promote development during early childhood, covering expenses for healthcare, early intervention programmes, childcare and preschool. When children are in school between the ages of 7–16, funds in Edusave are available to purchase educationally enriching programmes to complement schooling. From age 13 onwards, assets are accumulated in PSEAs for educational opportunities in adolescence and early adulthood.

Though the multiple asset-building policies target specific life stages (see Figure 1), the policies are also integrated to provide a system of asset building throughout childhood, and later linking to lifelong asset building in the CPF. As noted, unused balances in CDAs and Edusave are automatically rolled over into PSEAs at the relevant ages, which in turn roll over into the CPF if not fully used by age 30. In this fundamental sense, the various asset-building accounts could be described as a single lifelong account with specific and different uses at different life stages.

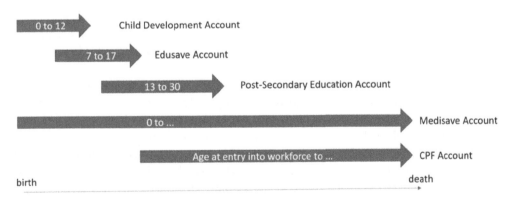

Figure 1. Singapore's asset-building accounts over the lifespan.

Universal eligibility and automatic enrolment

With various expansions and enhancements to asset-building policies since their inception, all Singaporean children are now eligible to participate. In addition, Medisave, Edusave and PSEAs are automatically opened upon birth registration or at relevant ages. For CDAs, parents must apply online with a participating bank around the time of birth of the child. However, they are not required to visit the bank in person. As such, though there is no automatic enrolment for the CDAs, application to enrol is hassle-free with minimal administrative barriers.

Universal eligibility and automatic enrolments are two necessary elements for a CDA policy to achieve universal participation (Clancy & Beverly, 2017). With universal eligibility, every child can be included in the policy; with automatic, opt-out enrolments, every child will be included, unless otherwise elected by the parents. One without the other may result in less than full participation in the policies, and the children excluded are likely to be disproportionately disadvantaged (Sherraden, Clancy, & Beverly, 2018). Reflecting on Singapore's asset-building accounts for children, there is near universal participation for the accounts with automatic enrolment. However, participation rates for CDAs are lower, with 3–5% of eligible children not having opened accounts (Singapore Ministry of Social and Family Development, 2014).

The lower participation rate for CDAs could be due to parents not being aware of the policy, and therefore unable to opt-in to enrol their children. In a study on the perceptions of and participation in CDAs among a small low-income sample receiving services at a Family Service Center, Han and Chia (2012) found that 35% of participants were not aware of the policy and hence did not open accounts for their children. Had automatic enrolment been in place for CDAs, this lack of awareness about the policy would have been a non-factor. As a clear lesson for every policymaker to consider, it is a fact that opt-in designs are never fully inclusive. Especially regarding children, there seems to be little benefit to an opt-in policy.

Substantial governmental investments and transfers

Distinctive in Singapore's asset-building policies is the substantial governmental investment and transfers into asset-building accounts, typically with automatic deposits. For example, in 2016, Singapore's government enhanced CDAs with an automatic initial deposit of S$3,000 for all newborns to kickstart for the accounts. This enhancement of the CDA, in and of itself, eclipses current asset-building policy for children in most other countries (Sherraden, 2016).

Along with the initial deposit into the CDA, each child can potentially receive an additional S$3,000, S$9,000 or S$15,000 in savings matches from private contributions into their CDAs, and another S$8,000 or S$10,000 in unrestricted cash, depending on their birth order, under the Baby Bonus Scheme. They also receive an initial deposit of S$4,000 in their Medisave accounts at birth, and upwards of S$2,500 in annual contributions into their Edusave accounts when they are in school. Overall, each child, depending on birth order, would receive between S$20,500 and S$34,500, assuming the full CDA/PSEA savings match cap is attained. If no private savings were deposited into CDAs, each child, depending on birth order, still receives between S$17,500 and S$19,500 in governmental transfers to their asset-building accounts. These calculations do not include the occasional top-ups from the government.

Despite these substantial government contributions, universal eligibility and automatic enrolments, not all children are participating in asset-building policies, specifically CDAs, equally. For example, Han and Chia (2012) found that only 32% of the low-income sample who opened CDAs for their children saved in those accounts, and on average, only S$125 was saved. Moreover, 5% of CDAs have accumulated no savings (Driscoll, 2016).

Recognising that some families, especially those with lower incomes, may not have the means to accumulate meaningful amounts in their accounts, the government restructured CDA benefits in 2016. Though the total CDA benefits remained the same, the benefits were broken down into two components: (1) the co-savings matches and (2) the S$3,000 CDA First Step grant, rather than just the co-savings matches previously. With the CDA First Step grant, children from lower income families now have S$3,000 to kickstart their accounts, whereas those from families with higher means continue to receive the same total amount of CDA benefits as before. And to further support lower income families, the occasional government top-ups to the different accounts are often pegged to household economic status, with children from lower income households receiving larger amounts in the top-ups. For example, in 2015, children aged 6 years and younger from lower income families received an additional S$600 in their CDAs, compared to S$300 for those from higher income households.

Constant evolution

The asset-building approach in Singapore is constantly evolving in response to inefficiencies and changing circumstances; the government is very open to information and areas for improvement. In the words of Singapore's Deputy Prime Minister Tharman Shanmugaratnam, 'the biggest mistake is to think "if it ain't broke, don't fix it"' (Teng, 2017).

For example, CDAs have undergone several enhancements since its inception in 2000. When first implemented, CDAs were open from birth until age 6, after which unused balances were transferred to PSEAs. Recognising that families needed more time to save and/or leverage accumulated funds, the government subsequently extended the accounts until the accountholder reaches age 12. A highly significant change to CDAs is inclusion of the policy to cover every Singaporean citizen child. Another significant change has been the restructuring of co-savings matches with the provision of the CDA First Step grant, designed to kickstart asset accumulation; especially important for lower income families who find it difficult to save.

Investment and potential for investment growth

As a whole, the integrated CDA platform in Singapore potentially provides a substantial resource pool for investments, and a fairly long time horizon of up to 30 years for investment growth. However, CDA policies are currently structured as savings accounts – or more accurately, interest-earning transactional accounts – with no other investment options. This severely limits the investment growth potential for the accounts, especially given the long investment time horizon. One area where the Singapore approach to CDAs could be improved would be to allow for some portion of the funds accumulated in CDAs and PSEAs to be invested in a selection of options with some exposure to bonds and equities to increase potential returns.

Conclusions

Singapore has by far the most extensive asset-building policies for children and youth in the world (Sherraden, 2016); therefore, the experiences of Singapore may be informative for other countries exploring and designing asset-building structures for children. Though these policy experiences may be in some ways unique to Singapore, some main themes are likely to apply in other settings. Policymakers in other countries may want consider modifications to fit their own circumstances.

First, in Singapore there is strong support for the various CDA policies, because asset building fits well within Singapore's established policy themes and values. In developing CDA policies elsewhere, governing authorities may consider how well asset-building policy aligns with national experiences, values and priorities. Alignment leads to support from the community, which is necessary for a CDA policy to be successful. Buy-in may be extensive, even across political differences. For example, in the United States, there is some measure of bipartisan support for CDAs as conservatives see CDAs as promoting individual responsibility, whereas progressives see CDAs as a platform to create opportunities for every child.

Second, one of the critiques of CDAs is that it is unrealistic to expect families to save for an uncertain event in the distant future when there are more immediate needs and concerns. For example, for a child to use the assets in a CDA for college tuition in the future, the child must first have resources available to pay for food, healthcare, books and to leverage developmental opportunities in early and middle childhood. Without investments in the present, there may not be a need for the resources in the future. However, well-designed policy can take this into account. It is not necessary for CDAs to focus on the future at the expense of the present, or vice versa. The CDA policies in Singapore strike a balance between current and future needs. This is somewhat different from CDA policies in the United States, where CDAs are often designed as long-term accounts for post-secondary education purposes. Each country must determine CDA priorities, and each country can and should look to other policy examples in this process.

Third, the policies in Singapore are designed with the principles of universality, automatic enrolments and automatic initial deposits to achieve maximum participation and benefits to all citizen children. Not all present at the outset, these design elements were introduced later in response to greater understanding and public support. Governments looking into introducing CDA policies may also consider starting with more basic designs, and expanding over time in step with the changing environment. In the same vein, asset-building policies in Singapore are continually being revised to remain relevant and effective. No policy is perfect, and constant refinements and enhancements are needed.

Looking ahead, one area of potential CDA revision and expansion in Singapore is the potential for inclusion of noncitizen children of Permanent Residents. Singapore has a large immigrant workforce, sometimes creating tensions in the community and in social policy. It is not clear that restricting social policy benefits to citizens is ideal. One opportunity for policy outreach to noncitizens would be support for the development of children. This could have positive payoffs in social harmony within Singapore, and at the same time contribute to positive social development, whether the children grow up to live in Singapore or elsewhere.

As the final and most important point, potential accumulation in the various CDA policies in Singapore is substantial enough to generate meaningful impacts on child and youth development. This is a lesson that other countries may want to learn. CDAs are not simply about having an account, but about developing each human being. Investments are required to make this successful, and Singapore is making these investments.

Disclosure statement

No potential conflict of interest was reported by the authors.

References

Clancy, M. M., & Beverly, S. G. (2017). *Statewide Child Development Account policies: Key design elements* (CSD Policy Report 17–30). St. Louis, MO: Center for Social Development, Washington University in St. Louis.

Curley, J., & Sherraden, M. (2000). Policy lessons from children's allowances for children's savings accounts. *Child Welfare, 79*(6), 661–687.

Driscoll, S. (2016, March 24). Singapore budget 2016: Parents to get $3,000 in child development account of babies born from March 24. *The Straits Times*. Retrieved from http://www.straitstimes.com/business/economy/singapore-budget-2016-parents-to-get-3000-in-child-development-account-of-babies

Han, C. H., & Chia, A. (2012). A preliminary study on parents savings in the child development account in Singapore. *Children and Youth Services Review, 34*(9), 1583–1589.

Haskins, R. (2011). Social policy in Singapore: A crucible of individual responsibility. *Social Genome Project Research*. Retrieved from https://www.brookings.edu/articles/social-policy-in-singapore-a-crucible-of-individual-responsibility/

Loke, V., & Cramer, R. (2009). *Singapore's Central Provident Fund: A national policy of life-long asset accounts* (New America Foundation Working Paper). Washington, D.C.: New America Foundation.

Loke, V., & Sherraden, M. (2009). Building assets from birth: A global comparison of child development account policies. *International Journal of Social Welfare, 18*(2), 119–129.

Loke, V., & Sherraden, M. (2015). *Building children's assets in Singapore: The beginning of a lifelong policy* (CSD Policy Brief 15–51). St. Louis, MO: Center for Social Development,

Washington University in St. Louis. Retrieved from https://csd.wustl.edu/Publications/Documents/PB15–51.pdf

Sherraden, M. (1991). *Assets and the poor*. Armonk, NY: M.E. Sharpe.

Sherraden, M. (2016). All babies building assets: Singapore expands child development accounts. Retrieved from https://csd.wustl.edu/newsroom/news/Pages/Singapore.CDAs.2016.aspx

Sherraden, M. (2018). Challenges in asset building in Singapore. In S. Vasoo & B. Singh (Eds.), *Critical issues in asset building in Singapore's development* (pp. 1–20). Singapore: World Scientific.

Sherraden, M., Cheng, L., Ssewamala, F., Kim, Y., Loke, V., Zou, L., … Han, C. H. (2018). International child development accounts. *Encyclopedia of Social Work*. doi:10.1093/acrefore/9780199975839.013.1261

Sherraden, M., Clancy, M. M., & Beverly, S. G. (2018). *Taking Child Development Accounts to scale: Ten key policy design elements* (CSD Policy Brief 18–08). St. Louis, MO: Center for Social Development, Washington Univeristy in St Louis. Retrieved from https://csd.wustl.edu/Publications/Documents/PB18–08.pdf

Sherraden, M., Nair, S., Vasoo, S., Liang, N. T., & Sherraden, M. S. (1995). Social policy based on assets: The impact of Singapore's central provident fund. *Asian Journal of Political Science, 3* (2), 112–133.

Singapore Government. (n.d.). Medisave grant for newborns. Retrieved from https://www.hey baby.sg/having-and-raising-children/medisave-grant-for-newborns

Singapore Ministry of Education. (2017). *The Education Endowment and Savings Schemes - Annual report for financial year 2016/2017*. Retrieved from https://www.moe.gov.sg/docs/default-source/document/initiatives/edusave/files/edusave-report-2016-amp-2017.pdf

Singapore Ministry of Education. (n.d.). Eligibility: Who is eligible for a PSEA? Retreived from https://www.moe.gov.sg/education/post-secondary/post-secondary-education-account/eligibility

Singapore Ministry of Finance. (2015). Budget 2015: families. Retrieved from https://www.singaporebudget.gov.sg/budget_2015/bib_pf

Singapore Ministry of Finance. (2018). Budget 2018 – Budget in brief. Retrieved from https://www.singaporebudget.gov.sg/data/budget_2018/download/FY2018_Budget_in_Brief_ENG.pdf

Singapore Ministry of Social and Family Development. (2014). Statistics of children without Child Development Account (CDA). Retrieved from https://www.msf.gov.sg/media-room/Pages/Statistics-of-children-without-Child-Development-Account-(CDA).aspx

Singapore Ministry of Social and Family Development. (2016). Opening speech by Mr Tan Chuan-Jin, minister for social and family development, at committee of supply, 2016 – Equal opportunities. Strong families. United country. Retrieved from http://www.nas.gov.sg/archivesonline/data/pdfdoc/20160412012/MSF%20COS%202016%20-%20OPENING%20SPEECH%20BY%20MINISTER%20TAN%20%28Media%29.pdf

Singapore Prime Minister's Office. (2008, August 20). Government doubles budget to provide more support for marriage and parenthood [Media release]. Retrieved from http://www.nas.gov.sg/archivesonline/data/pdfdoc/20080820988.pdf

Steering Group on Population. (2004, August 25). Singapore Government Media Release: New package of measures to support parenthood. Retrieved from http://www.nas.gov.sg/archiveson line/speeches/view-html?filename=2004082502.htm

Sung, J. (2006). *Explaining the economic success of Singapore: The developmental worker as the missing link*. Cheltenham, UK: Edward Elgar.

Tarmugi, A. (1995). Statement by Mr Abdullah Tarmugi, acting minister for community development at the world summit for social development, Copenhagen, Denmark, on 10 March 1995. Retrieved from http://www.un.org/documents/ga/conf166/gov/950310074254.htm

Teng, A. (2017, September 22). DPM Tharman on Singapore's education system: Biggest mistake is to think 'if it ain't broke, don't fix it'. *The Straits Times*. Retrieved from http://www.straitstimes.com/singapore/education/biggest-mistake-is-to-think-if-it-aint-broke-dont-fix-it

Vasoo, S., & Singh, B. (Eds.). (2018). *Critical issues in asset building in Singapore's development*. Singapore: World Scientific.

The Saving for Every Child Program in Israel: an overview of a universal asset-building policy

Michal Grinstein-Weiss, Olga Kondratjeva, Stephen P. Roll, Ofir Pinto and Daniel Gottlieb

ABSTRACT
In 2017, the Israeli government implemented a universal child development account programme – the Saving for Every Child Program (SECP) – which establishes a personal savings account for every Israeli child and provides monthly deposits until the child turns 18. The SECP has the potential to provide substantial assets when children reach adulthood, but the benefits depend on parents' investment choices. The unique programme's nature presents opportunities to learn from its implementation. This paper provides a comprehensive overview of the SECP, its legislative history, early findings from its implementation, and recommendations that may improve programme participation and outcomes across population groups.

Introduction

Among developed countries, Israel's rates of poverty and economic inequality are some of the highest (Milgrom & Bar-Levav, 2015; Organisation for Economic Co-operation and Development [OECD], 2017a, 2017b; National Insurance Institute [NII], 2017). At 18.6%, the overall poverty rate in Israel was the highest among the OECD countries in 2014 – the most recent year for which full data are available – and the youth poverty rate was the second highest at 24.3% (OECD, 2017b). The level of measured income inequality in Israel was also among the highest in OECD countries (NII, 2017; OECD, 2017a), with research indicating that wealth inequality in Israel may be higher than the level of income inequality (Milgrom & Bar-Levav, 2015).

To address these issues, Israeli policymakers have implemented a wide array of social welfare policies. Parents also receive additional income support through the Child Allowance programme, which provides between 150 NIS[1] and 189 NIS (between $40 and $51 USD as of January 2019 exchange rates) per child per month.

Israel's antipoverty programmes have traditionally supported income and consumption in poor households rather than asset-building and long-term investment behaviours. Distinguishing between income-support policies and asset-building policies is important, as changes in short- and long-term asset accumulation can have implications for household well-being that are distinct from changes in income or consumption (Sherraden, 1991). In the short term, having a modest amount of liquid assets can help buffer households against hardships (e.g. not being able to afford food, skipping bill payments) (Gjertson, 2016; McKernan, Ratcliffe, & Vinopal, 2009). In the long term, building assets can help families emerge from poverty, by enabling investments in housing and education.

To promote asset building, the Israeli government implemented a child development account (CDA) policy in January 2017. The programme developed as a result of this policy, called the Saving for Every Child Program (SECP), is universal; it automatically covers every Israeli child aged 18 or younger. The programme deposits a minimum of 50 NIS (around $13.5 USD) per month into accounts in the name of the child. Once enrolled, parents can both opt to transfer an additional 50 NIS per month from their Child Allowance benefits into the SECP accounts and choose from a range of low-yield savings accounts to high-yield investment accounts.

Though a number of countries have implemented CDAs – including Canada, Singapore, South Korea and many US states (Loke & Sherraden, 2009; Prosperity Now, 2017) – the universality, deposit structure and level of choice within the SECP make the Israeli policy unique. As such, the development, implementation and initial reception of the SECP presents a learning opportunity for researchers, policymakers and practitioners working on CDAs. This paper presents a comprehensive overview of the SECP, including its development through the policy process, its programme components and some initial results outlining how households are engaging with the programme. This paper also outlines several comprehensive recommendations that may potentially improve both household engagement with the programme and its long-term impacts on asset accumulation and economic mobility across income levels and ethnic groups.

Legislative background

Initial efforts to adopt a CDA policy in Israel can be traced to discussions in the early 2000s around creating regional Middle East Development Accounts – an idea that did not receive substantial support at the time (Sherraden et al., 2016). The proposal returned to the policy agenda after several years, when the Israeli government expressed its commitment to develop a savings account programme for children (Refaeli & Hermetz, 2018). The process of designing and adopting a national CDA policy began with a series of meetings between Israeli government officials and US policymakers and academics in 2009 and 2010.

In 2010, representatives from Israel's NII and the Ministry of Social Affairs and Social Services collaborated with academics and researchers to draft an initial proposal. The initial plan stressed the importance of asset accumulation and investments in child development as a means towards alleviating persistent poverty (Gottlieb & Toledano, 2010; Grinstein-Weiss, Gottlieb, & Sabah, 2010). It called for a universal, progressive CDA policy, with government matches on families' deposits, limits on the use of funds for prespecified purposes, and restrictions on the age at which funds would be available to beneficiaries. The proposal presented a design for a potential CDA policy and several incentive options to encourage savings behaviours among account holders (Grinstein-Weiss et al., 2010).

Following these discussions, a proposal for a nationwide CDA policy was introduced into Israel's parliament in 2010. After it was rejected, two policy developments contributed to the subsequent adoption of the bill. First, in August 2013, Child Allowance benefits were reduced by 13.6% compared to the previous year (NII, 2013). This decrease was expected to negatively and disproportionately affect families with a higher number of children, including the households of Arab Israelis and Ultra-Orthodox Jews (OECD, 2018). Second, a special committee – the Committee for the 'War Against Poverty' – was established in 2013 with a goal to improve economic conditions of the Israeli population (Gal & Madhala-Brik, 2016). This committee acknowledged the importance of asset building for children's long-term development and proposed a pilot child savings programme (Elalouf Committee, 2014), incorporating suggestions by Gottlieb and Toledano (2010) and Srulovici, Taylor, and Grinstein-Weiss (2012).

Despite this plan, there was no significant movement on the policy until 2015 when, shortly after parliamentary elections, it received overwhelming support from the majority of parliament members. The opposition leader and the coalition government agreed to enact the policy, and the Ultra-Orthodox political party – which had been pushing for an increase in Child Allowance benefits – agreed to integrate the bill into the new state budget (Grinstein-Weiss, Covington, Clancy, & Sherraden, 2016). The bill was signed into law in November 2015. The Israeli SECP went into effect on 1 January 2017, and Israel became the first country to have a CDA policy where the government provides automatic monthly deposits into savings or investment accounts for every child in the country (Sherraden et al., 2016).

Saving for Every Child Program (SECP) overview

The passage of the Israeli CDA policy led to the development and implementation of the SECP, which is administered by the NII. Through the SECP, the NII deposits 50 NIS into the account of every Israeli child aged younger than 18 years on a monthly basis. The programme is universal and automatically enrols children while allowing parents flexibility in managing their children's savings deposits.[2] In this section, we provide a detailed overview of the SECP's enrolment options, enrolment process, withdrawal limitations, bonuses and projected payouts.

Active and default enrolment options

Figure 1 provides a summary of the two enrolment choices available to parents: active or default. Parents who choose active enrolment can supplement the deposit amount and select the location of the SECP funds. In addition to the standard deposit amount of 50 NIS, parents can transfer an additional 50 NIS from their unrestricted monthly Child Allowance to the SECP account, for a total monthly deposit amount of 100 NIS. In essence, this choice involves shifting a portion of their monthly public support payments from current consumption (the Child Allowance) to future consumption (the SECP) for their child.[3]

Active enrolment also enables parents to select either a savings account or a variety of investment funds for their children's SECP funds. Funds deposited into savings accounts with fixed or variable interest will earn relatively low returns over the long

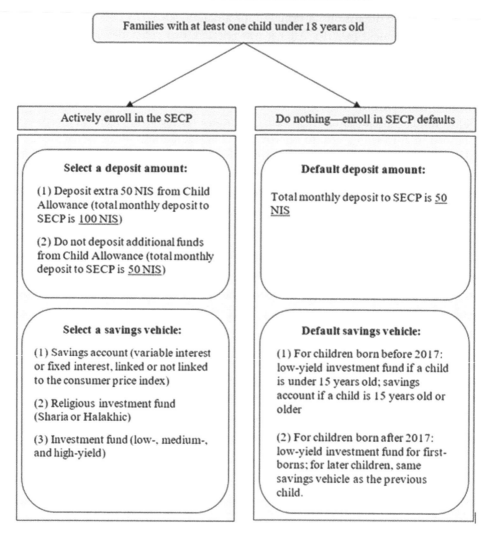

Figure 1. Structure of SECP enrolment choices.
Source: National Insurance Institute in Israel (2018).

run. Investment funds tend to have higher rates of return, which vary substantially depending on the fund. Parents who opt to invest in these funds can choose between low-, medium- and high-yield investment tracks, as well as religious investment accounts – either Sharia or Halakhic – that are compliant with Islamic or Jewish religious principles, respectively. These religious funds generally have lower rates of return. The average rates of return for different savings options, as of January 2019, were 9.07% for high-yield investment funds, 6.32% for medium-yield investment funds, 4.16% for Halakhic investment funds, 3.52% for low-yield investment funds, 1.20% for savings accounts, and –0.05% for Sharia-compliant investment funds.[4]

Children whose parents decide not to actively enrol or miss the 6-month active enrolment window are automatically enrolled into the SECP's default track. Under the default plan, the NII deposits a total of 50 NIS per month. The default savings vehicle was age-dependent for children born before the SECP went into effect on 1 January 2017: children under the age of 15 on this date had their deposits placed in a low-return investment fund, and children aged 15 or older had theirs deposited into a fixed-interest savings account. For children born after the SECP start date, the default savings vehicle depends on a child's birth order: their savings will be deposited into a low-return investment fund for firstborns, and other children will be enrolled in the same savings accounts as previous children in the household. Parents' previous choices about the transfer of additional 50 NIS from the Child Allowance for earlier children do not carry over to later children.

Online enrolment process

Families can enrol in the SECP online, over the phone, or in-person. Figure 2 illustrates how the choice between savings vehicles – investment funds or savings accounts – is presented to parents who actively enrol online. It demonstrates how the choice structure may promote decisions that enhance asset accumulation. On this screen, the upper panel (panel a) asks parents to specify whether they want to double their savings amount by transferring an extra 50 NIS from the Child Allowance to the SECP account. This option appears first and is automatically preselected, making it appear as the default choice. A brief explanation underneath emphasises that, by keeping deposits at 100 NIS per month, families will be able to save 1200 NIS per year. The lower panel (panel b) demonstrates how families can choose between different savings vehicles, with the investment fund option coming before the savings account option.

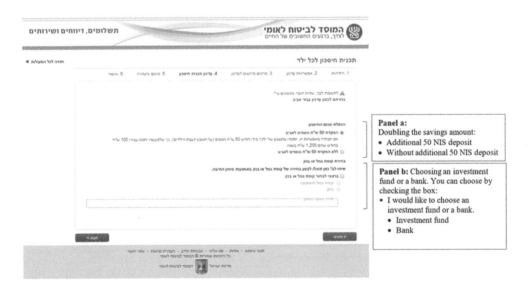

Figure 2. Online enrolment process, choosing deposit amount and savings vehicle.

Notes: Summarised translation from Hebrew to English is provided in boxes. Source: National Insurance Institute in Israel.

Parents also receive annual account statements that summarise the SECP account balances and benefits. As the SECP allows parents to change their selections for a deposit amount and a savings vehicle, these statements provide feedback that may help parents determine whether they have made appropriate decisions.

Withdrawal limitations

Except in cases of a child's severe illness or death, SECP savings can be withdrawn only after a child reaches 18 years of age. To withdraw funds before the age of 21, children must fill out withdrawal forms, obtain parental signatures and contact the bank or investment fund administering the SECP account. Parental approval is not needed to withdraw funds after the age of 21.[5] Though participants are encouraged to use the funds toward long-term investments such as homeownership or education, there are no specific restrictions on the use of funds.

Bonuses and projected pay out amounts

Several bonuses offered at different points in the child's life provide additional boosts in savings and may incentivise beneficiaries to keep their savings in SECP accounts for a longer period of time. Children born after 1 January 2017 are eligible for three bonuses: 251 NIS (approximately $68 USD) at the age of 3; 251 NIS at the age of 12 (for girls) or 13 (for boys); and 502 NIS (approximately $136 USD) at the age of 21.

Altogether, with regular investments throughout childhood and adolescence and the addition of bonuses, the payouts from this programme can be substantial, but they depend heavily on parents' investment choices. It is estimated that children whose parents make more conservative programme choices (50 NIS per month deposited in a savings account, with funds withdrawn at the age of 18) can expect to receive around 12,600 NIS, or enough to finance approximately 1 year of undergraduate education expenses. Children whose parents make the least conservative decisions (100 NIS per month deposited in a high-yield investment fund and no withdrawal until the age of 21) can expect around 72,700 NIS, or enough to cover over 5 years of college tuition, which is equivalent to financing at least a bachelor's degree in Israel (Grinstein-Weiss et al., 2018).

Summarising initial analyses of SECP enrolment

Recent work by Grinstein-Weiss et al. (2018) assesses the early SECP participation patterns of Israeli households. Using an administrative data set provided by the NII containing demographic, financial and SECP enrolment records on approximately 3.1 million Israeli children in 1.3 million households, this study found:

(1) Almost 65% of Israeli households actively enrolled in the programme over the first 6 months of the SECP's existence. Of these, nearly 65% opted to shift 50 NIS from their Child Allowance into their SECP account and 60% deposited their funds into an investment account rather than a savings account.

(2) Households with young children or with high numbers of children tended to actively enrol at higher rates and deposit to investment funds at higher rates.

However, households with high numbers of children were less likely to transfer the additional 50 NIS from their Child Allowance.

(3) Lower wage households, households with low educational attainment and Arab Israeli households tended to engage with the programme less, controlling for other observable demographic and financial factors. These groups actively enrolled at lower rates, and were less likely to deposit the additional 50 NIS into their SECP account or deposit to an investment fund than households with higher household wages, higher educational attainment and Non-Ultra-Orthodox Jews.

(4) There is suggestive evidence that a targeted outreach campaign to Ultra-Orthodox communities was effective. Early in the SECP's implementation, active enrolment rates in this population were very low. However, immediately following discussions between the NII and leading Ultra-Orthodox rabbis, as well as a targeted advertising campaign, SECP enrolment rates rose rapidly towards the end of the initial enrolment period and eventually exceeded the enrolment rates of Non-Ultra-Orthodox Jews. However, Ultra-Orthodox Jews were less likely to deposit an additional 50 NIS into their SECP funds than Non-Ultra-Orthodox Jews, and though they selected investment funds at a higher rate, they tended to choose lower yield Halakhic investment funds.

The evidence points to high levels of initial household engagement with the SECP, but also demonstrates that many of the households who could derive the most benefit from this programme (e.g. those with low incomes, low educational attainment or who are from economically vulnerable ethnic minority groups) engage at lower levels and in ways that will likely lead to lower rates of asset accumulation over their children's lives.

Policy recommendations

Though the early results are encouraging, a number of policy design and implementation considerations may further affect the SECP's long-term success and improve its impact on the financial lives of Israeli households. This section outlines a number of recommendations Israeli policymakers could consider for the SECP.[6]

Incorporate a progressive deposit structure

Though the SECP is likely to increase the overall level of assets available to all Israeli children upon reaching adulthood, the evidence from early enrolment trends indicates that the structure of the Israel's CDA policy may exacerbate existing levels of wealth inequality in Israel. In the first 6 months of the SECP's implementation, non-minority, higher income and more educated households tended to invest their funds in ways that would lead to higher asset accumulation than more economically vulnerable and minority groups (Grinstein-Weiss et al., 2018). This pattern is not unique to Israeli CDA policy – other countries' CDA policies also tend to engender higher participation levels from relatively affluent segments of the population (Han & Chia, 2012; Huang, Beverly, Clancy, Lassar, & Sherraden, 2013; Imbeau, 2015; Kempson, Finney, & Davies, 2011). However, the universality of the SECP makes it well-positioned to address this disparity in long-term asset accumulation. As every child is covered by the policy, any changes to the deposit structure will affect the entire population regardless of economic condition, and not just those who opt-in. Thus, introducing a progressive deposit structure may represent a means of reducing wealth inequality in Israel.[7]

This progressive structure could take a number of forms. First, the government could provide an additional savings match for low-income households who opt to transfer funds from the Child Allowance to their SECP account. From a household budgeting perspective, the decision to forgo the unrestricted funds of the Child Allowance to save in the SECP account is likely more difficult for lower income households than it is for higher income households. Providing a matching deposit for lower income households that save additional funds would recognise that difficulty and further promote investment behaviours in low-income households.

Second, low-income households could receive an initial seed deposit into their account that would grow over the lifespan of the account. This approach would combine the recurring deposit structure of the SECP with the upfront investment structure of SEED OK or proposed 'baby bond' programmes (Beverly, Clancy, & Sherraden, 2016; Darity & Hamilton, 2012), and could build on the additional deposits made into the SECP at different points in the child's life.

Third, increasing the recurring deposit amounts for low-income households would be sensitive to changes in household income over the life of the child – parents whose incomes fell after the birth of a child would benefit from increased deposit amounts, whereas parents whose incomes rose after the birth of a child would have their deposit amounts unchanged.

Alter the timing of bonuses

Currently, SECP recipients have the potential to receive three additional bonus payments through the programme at the age of 3, 12 or 13 (for girls and boys, respectively), and 21 (if they keep their funds in their account). Shifting the timing of these bonuses would be a straightforward way of altering the SECP structure to further promote asset building. Though the conditional payment at 21 may promote saving for a longer period and allow the SECP funds to grow, the earlier payments do not necessarily incentivise additional saving. Shifting these payments to a single seed deposit made at birth would allow parents to earn interest for several more years. If 502 NIS were deposited at birth rather than split between early childhood and adolescence, this could result in an additional asset accumulation of 1139 NIS (if withdrawn at the age of 18) to 1494 NIS (if withdrawn at the age of 21).[8]

Pair the programme with financial education or financial capability programmes

Given that the SECP funds are unrestricted and may develop into a substantial amount over 18 to 21 years (Grinstein-Weiss et al., 2018), it is important to provide education, training and guidance for children around how to use these funds in ways that will improve their long-term well-being. In many ways, schools provide a promising setting for financial training initiatives that complement the SECP: They are universally available and can provide multiple educational interventions around the usage of SECP funds tailored to different ages, and can potentially integrate parents into the discussion. Providing financial education programmes during military service, which is mandatory for most Israelis (there are exceptions based primarily around religious or ethnic considerations), also presents an opportunity.

The design of SECP-focused financial education programmes is important. Meta-analyses of general financial education programmes (Fernandes, Lynch, & Netemeyer, 2014; Miller, Reichelstein, Salas, & Zia, 2015) have found very limited evidence of their impact on downstream financial behaviours; the measured impacts of financial education decay rapidly. At the same time, Fernandes et al. (2014) show that 'just-in-time' education delivered around key financial moments (e.g. purchasing a house, taking on student debt) may make an impact on financial decisions. These findings have several implications for the integration of SECP-based financial education into school or military settings. First, at a minimum, educational efforts should be focused on points where SECP beneficiaries will be making decisions on how to use their funds. In school settings, financial education could occur at the age of 18 when children can withdraw their funds with parental permission; in the military, it could be towards the end of beneficiaries' service term, when they are approaching the age at which they can access the funds without parental approval. Second, education delivered earlier in children's lives should focus on concrete behaviours and actions. Such efforts could educate parents and children on the implications of different SECP choices, encouraging parents to change their investment decisions to increase asset accumulation over time. Third, financial capability programmes that provide regular feedback and are tailored to the individual needs of participants, such as financial coaching programmes (Collins & O'Rourke, 2010), may be more effective than general financial education. Financial coaching programmes have been shown to affect a wide array of financial outcomes (Theodos, Stacy, & Daniels, 2018), and can potentially be targeted towards military service members, as have been done in the United States (Consumer Financial Protection Bureau, 2015).

Restrict the use of SECP funds to investment purposes

Currently, SECP participants do not face any restrictions on how to use the funds. This separates the current incarnation of Israel's CDA policy from many other CDA policies (Loke & Sherraden, 2009), and from the early policy proposals for Israeli CDAs (Gottlieb & Toledano, 2010; Grinstein-Weiss et al., 2010; Srulovici et al., 2012) – which restrict funds to educational expenses, home purchases or starting a business. Though it is plausible that many SECP recipients will use these funds for investments to enhance their economic mobility, many may spend them on vacations or expensive goods.

There is limited research on the impact of fund restrictions for CDAs, but evidence from cash transfer programmes suggests that fund restrictions may improve long-term economic mobility. Baird, Ferreira, Özler, and Woolcock (2014) found that restricted cash transfer programmes were more effective than unrestricted programmes at increasing school enrolment – particularly in cases where the conditions were explicit and compliance was strongly enforced. This indicates that restricting the SECP funds to purposes explicitly oriented towards enhancing economic mobility (e.g. investments in education, certain capital assets) may enhance the programmes long-term impacts on children's well-being and economic outcomes.

Identify additional opportunities to effectively promote enrolment

Identifying additional touchpoints with parents can promote enrolment in the SECP. The current standard outreach method involves sending letters to families after the birth of a child, but additional points of contact are necessary to further encourage programme enrolment. For example, hospitals and vaccination clinics could provide new parents with take-home information sheets on SECP enrolment, provide ways to enrol during the vaccination process (e.g. tablets or computers), and incorporate SECP discussions into the standard patient-intake procedure. Moreover, parents currently receive a yearly benefit statement for the SECP, which could be modified to outline how much families are currently projected to receive under the SECP and how much they could receive if they changed their enrolment decisions.

Target outreach to economically vulnerable populations

Early analyses of the SECP (Grinstein-Weiss et al., 2018) show a close link between targeted outreach to the Ultra-Orthodox communities (by working closely with Rabbinical authorities) and Ultra-Orthodox households actively engaging in the programme, which indicates that public outreach may influence programme enrolment. These results are encouraging as Ultra-Orthodox households tend to report higher levels of economic hardship than the general population (Lewin & Stier, 2017). However, Arab Israelis – a group with similar levels of economic vulnerability to Ultra-Orthodox Jews (National Insurance Institute of Israel, 2017) – engaged with the programme at much lower rates than Ultra-Orthodox and Non-Ultra-Orthodox Jews. Similarly, households with lower incomes or lower educational attainment tended to engage in the SECP at much lower rates and invest in lower yield savings vehicles, even when controlling for other demographic and financial characteristics.

Finding ways of reaching out to these groups to promote effective asset-building investment behaviours is essential to address issues of economic inequality. Though there is evidence that more targeted outreach campaigns, like those targeting Ultra-Orthodox communities, can influence enrolment behaviours, more generalised outreach campaigns targeting social service offices, public hospitals and vaccination clinics may also be effective in reaching low-income households.

These general outreach efforts could be complemented by targeted outreach to specific economically vulnerable communities (e.g. Arab Israelis). It will be important to work with religious leaders, employers, local non-profits and other government agencies embedded in these communities to find ways of increasing household engagement with the SECP. Doing so will not only provide channels into these communities, but will also incorporate the expertise of these community stakeholders into any outreach campaign. It may also be beneficial to better leverage social media to promote the programme in a way that reaches communities that exhibit low enrolment rates – for example, promoting the programme on city- or neighbourhood-specific social media in geographies with low enrolment rates. This approach will allow for direct communication with community members themselves and has the potential to reach these communities in way that traditional media approaches might not. Finally, better integration of additional languages into SECP-related material – for example, the NII's letters to new parents and online enrolment forms are currently only offered in Hebrew – may enhance Arab Israelis' and other minority groups' understanding of and engagement with the programme.

Test behavioural economics approaches to improve enrolment and impact

Behavioural economics research has demonstrated how simple changes to decision environments can substantially affect individual decision-making. These behavioural interventions can include changing default decisions (e.g. Madrian & Shea, 2001), making certain options more salient (e.g. Grinstein-Weiss et al., 2017a), providing reminders (e.g. Karlan, McConnell, Mullainathan, & Zinman, 2016), 'anchoring' decisions through the use of suggested values (e.g. Grinstein-Weiss, Russell, Gale, Key, & Ariely, 2017b) or changing the content of messages (e.g. Cialdini, 2003). Whereas the SECP's existing behavioural design choices (see Figure 2) can nudge households into selections that increase their children's asset accumulation over time, there are other further opportunities to incorporate behavioural economics into the SECP's design.

Additionally, modifying existing modes of communication (such as letters or websites) with common behavioural economics techniques, such as increasing the salience of the potential benefits of the programme (e.g. Bhargava & Manoli, 2015), leveraging social norms around programme participation (e.g. Hallsworth, List, Metcalfe, & Vlaev, 2017) and cuing households to think about the future (e.g. Hershfield et al., 2011), may increase active enrolment and encourage increased savings deposits. Incorporating text- or social media-based reminders for households to enrol in the programme could further complement existing modes of communication.

Conclusion

The universal Israeli SECP provides a substantial base of assets for Israeli children upon their entering adulthood. Early analyses of the SECP are encouraging, as a majority of Israeli households with children opt to actively engage with the programme and, of these, a majority opt to make an additional monthly savings deposit for their children. However, further research is needed to understand the programme impacts on household behaviours, child well-being, and economic inequality, and to help policymakers further optimise household savings within the programme and promote economic mobility when beneficiaries enter adulthood.

Notes

1. Israeli New Shekel.
2. This discussion relies on information from the NII (https://hly.gov.il/default.html).
3. This would reduce the Child Allowance payments from 150 NIS to 100 NIS or from 189 NIS to 139 NIS, depending on family size.
4. Because the SECP assumes long-term investments for the period of 18 years, we assume that each account is associated with similarly low levels of risk in the long run. In the short run, the levels of potential risks may correspond to the expected rates of return: savings accounts are associated with lower risks, and low-, medium- and high-yield investment accounts are associated with low, medium and high short-term risks, respectively. The estimates assume normal market conditions and use information about examples of

investment funds provided by the NII (https://hly.gov.il/). The estimated annual percentage rates are subject to change according to market conditions.

5. Account management fees are covered by the NII until beneficiaries reach 21 years of age. Account holders are responsible for paying taxes on the capital gains. For those who will decide to keep the funds until they retire and use them after retirement, the savings will be tax-exempt.

6. Grinstein-Weiss et al. (2016) discusses several of these recommendations, including providing financial education around SECP accounts in school settings and making the accounts progressive.

7. An array of potential progressive programme structures are outlined in Gal, Madhala-Brik, Grinstein-Weiss, and Covington (2016), Grinstein-Weiss et al. (2010) and Gottlieb and Toledano (2010).

8. Assuming a 9.07% rate of return on the high-yield investment track, reported as of January 2019.

Disclosure statement

No potential conflict of interest was reported by the authors.

References

Baird, S., Ferreira, F. H., Özler, B., & Woolcock, M. (2014). Conditional, unconditional and everything in between: A systematic review of the effects of cash transfer programmes on schooling outcomes. *Journal of Development Effectiveness*, 6(1), 1–43.

Beverly, S. G., Clancy, M. M., & Sherraden, M. (2016). *Universal accounts at birth: Results from SEED for Oklahoma kids*. (CSD Research Summary No. 16–07). St. Louis, MO: Washington University, Center for Social Development.

Bhargava, S., & Manoli, D. (2015). Psychological frictions and the incomplete take-up of social benefits: Evidence from an IRS field experiment. *American Economic Review*, *105*(11), 3489–3529.

Cialdini, R. B. (2003). Crafting normative messages to protect the environment. *Current Directions in Psychological Science*, *12*(4), 105–109.

Collins, J. M., & O'Rourke, C. M. (2010). Financial education and counseling – Still holding promise. *Journal of Consumer Affairs*, *44*(3), 483–498.

Consumer Financial Protection Bureau. (2015, May 20). *CFPB launches financial coaching initiative*. Retrieved from https://www.consumerfinance.gov/about-us/newsroom/cfpb-launches-financial-coaching-initiative/.

Darity, W., Jr., & Hamilton, D. (2012). Bold policies for economic justice. *The Review of Black Political Economy*, *39*(1), 79–85.

Elalouf Committee. (2014, July). *Report by the Israel committee for the war against poverty. Part 1: Plenary report* (Plenary Report). Retrieved from https://brookdale.jdc.org.il/wp-content/uploads/2014/07/The-War-against-Poverty.pdf

Fernandes, D., Lynch, J. G., Jr., & Netemeyer, R. G. (2014). Financial literacy, financial education, and downstream financial behaviors. *Management Science*, *60*(8), 1861–1883.

Gal, J., & Madhala-Brik, S. (2016, November) *Implementation of the Elalouf committee recommendations: The state of affairs.* (Policy Brief). Jerusalem, Israel: Taub Center for Social Policy Studies in Israel.

Gal, J., Madhala-Brik, S., Grinstein-Weiss, M., & Covington, M. (2016, July). *Child development accounts in Israel: Background and review of options.* Jerusalem, Israel: Taub Center for Social Policy Studies in Israel.

Gjertson, L. (2016). Emergency saving and household hardship. *Journal of Family and Economic Issues*, *37*(1), 1–17.

Gottlieb, D., & Toledano, E. (2010). A child empowerment grant – A policy proposal for a CDA. *Policy Proposal*, pp. 1–5 (in Hebrew). Retrieved from: https://www.btl.gov.il/Publications/more_publications/Documents/haazama.pdf

Grinstein-Weiss, M., Covington, M., Clancy, M. M., & Sherraden, M. (2016, April). *A savings account for every child born in Israel: Recommendations for program implementation.* (CSD Policy Brief No. 16–11). St. Louis, MO: Washington University, Center for Social Development.

Grinstein-Weiss, M., Cryder, C., Despard, M. R., Perantie, D. C., Oliphant, J. E., & Ariely, D. (2017a). The role of choice architecture in promoting saving at tax time: Evidence from a large-scale field experiment. *Behavioral Science & Policy*, *3*(2), 21–38.

Grinstein-Weiss, M., Gottlieb, D., & Sabah, Y. (2010). Child development accounts in Israel: Toward a new policy. *Policy white paper*. Jerusalem, Israel: Prepared for the Ministry of Welfare and Social Services.

Grinstein-Weiss, M., Pinto, O., Kondratjeva, O., Roll, S., Bufe, S., Barkali, N., & Gottlieb, D. (2018, July). *How do households choose to invest in a universal child savings program? Evidence from Israel.* Paper session presented at the meeting of Association for Public Policy Analysis and Management International Conference, Mexico City, Mexico.

Grinstein-Weiss, M., Russell, B. D., Gale, W. G., Key, C., & Ariely, D. (2017b). Behavioral interventions to increase tax-time saving: Evidence from a national randomized trial. *Journal of Consumer Affairs*, *51*(1), 3–26.

Hallsworth, M., List, J. A., Metcalfe, R. D., & Vlaev, I. (2017). The behavioralist as tax collector: Using natural field experiments to enhance tax compliance. *Journal of Public Economics*, *148*, 14–31.

Han, C.-K., & Chia, A. (2012). A preliminary study on parents saving in the child development account in Singapore. *Children and Youth Services Review*, *34*(9), 1583–1589.

Hershfield, H. E., Goldstein, D. G., Sharpe, W. F., Fox, J., Yeykelis, L., Carstensen, L. L., & Bailenson, J. N. (2011). Increasing saving behavior through age-progressed renderings of the future self. *Journal of Marketing Research*, *48*(SPL), S23–S37.

Huang, J., Beverly, S., Clancy, M., Lassar, T., & Sherraden, M. (2013). Early program enrollment in a statewide child development account program. *Journal of Policy Practice, 12*(1), 62–81.

Imbeau, E. (2015). *Analysis of the Canada education savings program participation and expenditures for different income groups.* Employment and Social Development of Canada. Retrieved from http://publications.gc.ca/collections/collection_2017/edsc-esdc/Em20-63-2017-eng.pdf

Karlan, D., McConnell, M., Mullainathan, S., & Zinman, J. (2016). Getting to the top of mind: How reminders increase saving. *Management Science, 62*(12), 3393–3411.

Kempson, E., Finney, A., & Davies, S. (2011). *The child trust fund: Findings from the wave 2 evaluation* (HM Revenue and Customs Research Report 143). Personal Finance Research Centre, University of Bristol. Retrieved from https://revenuebenefits.org.uk/pdf/report143.pdf

Lewin, A. C., & Stier, H. (2017). The experience of material and emotional hardship in Israel: Do some groups cope better than others? *Social Indicators Research, 134*(1), 385–402.

Loke, V., & Sherraden, M. (2009). Building assets from birth: A global comparison of child development account policies. *International Journal of Social Welfare, 18*, 119–129.

Madrian, B. C., & Shea, D. F. (2001). The power of suggestion: Inertia in 401(k) participation and savings behavior. *The Quarterly Journal of Economics, 116*(4), 1149–1187.

McKernan, S.-M., Ratcliffe, C., & Vinopal, K. (2009). *Do assets help families cope with adverse events?* Perspectives on Low-Income Working Families Brief 10. Washington, DC: Urban Institute.

Milgrom, M., & Bar-Levav, G. (2015). *The distribution of wealth in Israel.* Tel Aviv, Israel: The Institute for Structural Reforms.

Miller, M., Reichelstein, J., Salas, C., & Zia, B. (2015). Can you help someone become financially capable? A meta-analysis of the literature. *The World Bank Research Observer, 30*(2), 220–246.

National Insurance Institute in Israel. (2018). *Savings per child.* Retrieved from https://hly.gov.il/default.html.

National Insurance Institute of Israel. (2013). *Annual report. Chapter 3: Benefits: Children insurance* (Annual Report). Retrieved from https://www.btl.gov.il/English%20Homepage/Publications/AnnualSurvey/2013/Documents/Annual%20Report%202013.pdf.

National Insurance Institute of Israel. (2017). *Poverty and social gaps in 2016, annual report.* Retrieved from https://www.btl.gov.il/English%20Homepage/Publications/Poverty_Report/Documents/oni2016-e.pdf.

OECD. (2017a). *Income inequality* (indicator). doi:10.1787/459aa7f1-en

OECD (2017b), *Poverty rate* (indicator). doi:10.1787/0fe1315d-en

Organization for Economic Cooperation and Development (OECD). (2018, March). *OECD economic surveys: Israel 2018.* Paris: OECD Publishing. doi:10.1787/eco_surveys-isr-2018-en

Prosperity Now. (2017, August). Invest in every child's future with children's savings accounts. Retrieved from https://prosperitynow.org/resources/state-local-csa-overview-invest-every-childs-future-childrens-savings-accounts.

Refaeli, T., & Hermetz, S. (2018). *Child development aaccounts in Israel as a tool for reducing inter-generational poverty: A comparative study of international programs and analysis of the policy development in Israel.* Beer-Sheva: Ben Gurion University.

Sherraden, M. (1991). *Assets and the poor: A new American welfare policy.* New York: ME Sharpe.

Sherraden, M., Cheng, L.-C., Ssewamala, F. M., Kim, Y., Loke, V., Zou, L., ... Han, C.-K. (2016). International child development accounts. *CSD Working paper No. 16–48.* St. Louis, MO: Washington University, Center for Social Development.

Srulovici, E., Taylor, A., & Grinstein-Weiss, M. (2012). Asset building programs and policies: Applications for at-risk youth in Israel. *Commissioned policy paper for the Israel Ministry of Social Welfare.*

Theodos, B., Stacy, C. P., & Daniels, R. (2018). Client led coaching: A random assignment evaluation of the impacts of financial coaching programs. *Journal of Economic Behavior and Organization, 155*, 140–158.

Impacts of child development accounts on parenting practices: evidence from a randomised statewide experiment

Jin Huang, Yunju Nam, Michael Sherraden and Margaret Clancy

ABSTRACT
This study examines the impact of Child Development Accounts (CDAs) on parenting practices of mothers with young children in a statewide randomised experiment conducted in the United States. The experiment included 2704 primary caregivers of children born in Oklahoma during 2007: 1358 were randomly assigned to the treatment group and 1346 to the control group. Structural equation modelling suggests that the punitive-parenting score among treatment participants was .12 standard deviations smaller than that among control participants ($p < .05$). Findings indicate that CDAs reduce punitive parenting, and may serve as an additional tool for positive parent–child interactions.

Parenting practices influence child functioning (Shonkoff & Phillips, 2000). These practices comprise parental attitudes and patterned behaviours that define the parent–child relationship, including parental support and involvement, structure, positive discipline, psychological control, psychical punishment and other behaviours (Darling & Steinberg, 1993). Through appropriate direction, monitoring, and disciplinary efforts in the context of warm and supportive parent–child interactions, effective parenting practices can encourage self-control and responsible behaviours in children (Aunola & Nurmi, 2005; Gershoff, 2002). In contrast, inappropriate parenting behaviours can be a risk factor in children's development (Capaldi, Chamberlain, & Patterson, 1997; Gershoff, 2002). These typically involve several, often correlated, aspects of parenting, including low warmth and low positivity, noncontingent and harsh punishment and lack of supervision (Patterson, 2002).

Parenting practices are determined by numerous factors (Verhoeven, Junger, Van Aken, Deković, & Van Aken, 2007), which may be categorised into different domains within an ecological framework, such as parental characteristics, family context and social context. Parental characteristics include parental personality (e.g. extraversion, agreeableness, emotional stability), parenting cognition and skills, level of parental education, physical and mental health and other attributes. The family context domain consists of socioeconomic status (e.g. income, wealth), the marital relationship, children's characteristics (e.g. temperament), kinship support and intergenerationally transmitting parenting tradition. Social context (Belsky & Jaffee, 2006) includes support or stress from institutions related to child-rearing (e.g. availability of child care, parenting training, child tax credit), work and social relationships and cultural values and norms related to parenting.

Numerous initiatives to improve parenting practices attempt to modify parental behaviours and attitudes by educating caregivers about child development, parenting skills, anger management and stress-reduction techniques (Chaffin & Friedrich, 2004; MacLeod & Nelson, 2000; Segal, Opie, & Dalziel, 2012; Thomlison, 2004). In recognition that some risk factors for punitive parenting are beyond parental characteristics and control of caregivers, some recent programmes have paid attention to social, economic and cultural contexts in which parents live.

Child developmental accounts and parenting practices

A risk factor for child maltreatment, economic deprivation affects the quality of the child–caregiver relationship (Elder, Eccles, Ardelt, & Lord, 1995; Thomlison, 2004). However, little research has considered how an economic intervention might affect parenting practices.

This study seeks to fill this gap using data from SEED for Oklahoma Kids (SEED OK), a randomised policy experiment of universal and progressive Child Development Accounts (CDAs) in Oklahoma. Child Development Accounts are savings or investment accounts that provide financial access, information, subsidies, and incentives to encourage lifelong asset accumulation and to promote child development (e.g. Sherraden, 1991). Accumulated savings and financial assets in CDAs are usually intended to finance postsecondary education (Meyer, Masa, & Zimmerman, 2010).

Different from parent-training programmes and early-childhood education, CDAs provide no direct intervention on parenting practices. Nevertheless, CDAs may influence parenting practices. As CDAs promote asset holding for children (Nam, Kim, Clancy, & Zager, 2013), they may in turn also affect the attitudes and behaviours of parents. More specifically, CDAs may increase parents' perceived levels of economic safety, enhance their optimism concerning the long-term development of their child, improve parents' mental health and, therefore, reduce negative impacts of mental health conditions on parenting. Holding assets raise parents' expectations for their children's college education; therefore, they may also improve parenting behaviours (Zhan & Sherraden, 2003). In particular, CDAs help to reduce depressive symptoms of mothers with young children (Huang, Sherraden, Kim, & Clancy, 2014; Huang, Sherraden, & Purnell, 2014; Kim, Sherraden, Huang, & Clancy, 2015).

The premise that holding assets benefits parenting practices and child development is an expansion of the linkage between income and child development (Linver, Brooks-Gunn, & Kohen, 2002). Two mechanisms—the family stress model and the investment model—explain the association between income and child development (Linver et al., 2002). The family stress model identifies maternal emotional distress (e.g. depressive symptoms) and parenting behaviours (e.g. positive and punitive parenting) as mediators in the relationship between income and child behaviour. The investment model identifies a cognitively stimulating home environment as a mediator. We suggest that these two mechanisms can also explain asset holding's impact on parenting practices.

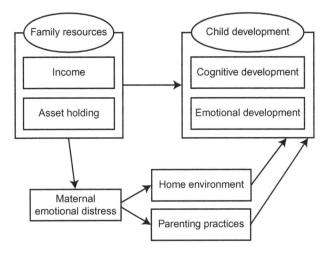

Figure 1. Theoretical model for asset effects on parenting practices: The family stress model and the investment model.

Figure 1 illustrates this proposition, which is similar to the theoretical framework that (Linver et al., 2002) presented for the income–child development link. We expand the framework to include *assets* as a type of family economic resource generated through CDAs.

The SEED OK CDA experiment

The SEED OK experiment is a statewide policy test designed to examine whether CDAs can successfully reach the universal population at birth, encourage asset accumulation among parents and children, and improve the attitudes and behaviours of parents and children. The SEED OK intervention was designed to pair with and adapt the centralised account structure of a state's tax-advantaged college savings plans (also known as 529 plans; U.S. Department of the Treasury, 2009).

Built on the 529 Plan's account structure, the SEED OK experiment drew a probability sample of 7328 infants from children born in Oklahoma in 2007. The caregivers of 2704 of the 7328 infants (37%) participated in the experiment and completed the baseline survey. More than 99% of these caregivers were mothers of the children identified in the sampling frame. The terms *treatment children* and *control children* refer to children whose primary caregivers were assigned to the respective groups. Participants who completed the baseline survey were randomly assigned into the treatment group (*n* = 1358) and the control group (*n* = 1346). A follow-up survey was conducted in 2011.

The SEED OK experiment offered three financial interventions to treatment mothers (see Figure 2). Details on the experiment and intervention components can be found in (Clancy, Beverly, Sherraden, & Huang, 2016). First, the Oklahoma treasurer's office automatically opened a *state-owned* OK 529 Plan account for treatment children and deposited $1000 of SEED OK funds into each account. Second, the SEED OK experiment encouraged treatment mothers to open and make deposits into their own

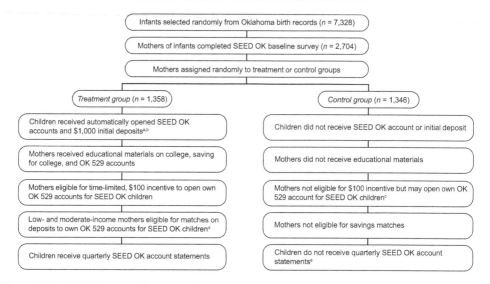

Figure 2. Study design, enrollment and retention for SEED OK participants.

participant-owned OK 529 Plan accounts by offering a $100 initial contribution. Third, the experiment offered low- and moderate-income treatment households savings matches for deposits made into the participant-owned OK 529 Plan accounts between 1 January 2008 and 31 December 2011. Participants in the control group were eligible to open a participant-owned OK 529 Plan account. However, they did not receive any of the intervention components.

Impacts of the SEED OK CDA on financial and nonfinancial outcomes

SEED OK CDAs have positive financial outcomes—including the holding of asset-building accounts, total assets and individual deposits in these accounts—for families in the treatment group (Beverly, Kim, Sherraden, Nam, & Clancy, 2015; Nam et al., 2013; Sherraden et al., 2015). Nearly 100% of the treatment families have automatic state-owned accounts. SEED OK CDAs also generate positive nonfinancial outcomes on parental educational expectations (Kim et al., 2015), mothers' mental health (Huang, Sherraden, & Purnell, 2014), and children's social–emotional development (Huang, Sherraden, Kim, & Clancy, 2014).

In particular, Nam, Wikoff, and Sherraden (2014) examined whether exposure to CDAs affected parental stress and six indicators of parenting; results identified that, on average, the number of times that treatment mothers screamed at their children in the 3 days prior to survey was significantly lower than the number of times that control mothers did so. Although the study by Nam et al. (2014) provided important insights in CDA effects on parenting practices, it had limitations. First, it assessed effects on individual parenting indicators separately, but a latent measure of parenting practices based on confirmatory factory analysis (CFA) might have been more reliable and had greater validity (Kline, 2011). Second, the three count variables that Nam et al. (2014) used to measure punitive parenting were highly skewed—a high proportion of mothers reported no punitive practices during the assessed period—and could be better modelled in Poisson regression. We reanalysed the association between the SEED OK experiment's CDA intervention and such practices. In particular, we used CFA to generate two latent measures of parenting practices (i.e. positive parenting and punitive parenting) from six parenting indicators, and we applied Poisson regression to define the latent punitive-parenting variable's relationships with the three count items.

Impacts of SEED OK research on state and national policy

SEED OK research has informed design and implementation of new CDA policies, and made existing policies more inclusive, effective, and sustainable. For example, in 2008, Maine created a CDA programme, and began offering $500 for future college expenses to every state resident new-born enrolled in the state's 529 plan before the child's first birthday. Since 2014, the Maine CDA programme automatically enrols all Maine newborns to receive the $500 grant. SEED OK research directly influenced the decision to adopt an opt-out structure, and Maine now has the first universal, statewide, at-birth CDA policy in the nation (Clancy & Sherraden, 2014). SEED OK research has also informed several other states' CDA initiatives, such as those in Connecticut, Rhode Island, and Nevada.

At the federal level, CDAs have been proposed several times, most prominently through the America Saving for Personal Investment, Retirement, and Education (ASPIRE) Act (New America Foundation, 2013). These policy discussions have recently been renewed (King, 2014), and researchers at the Center for Social Development are advising key staff in Congressional committees in which CDAs are being considered. SEED OK research will play an important role in federal initiatives to make 529 policies more inclusive.

Methods

Data and sample

Built on previous research from the SEED OK experiment, this study examines the potential impacts of the CDAs on parents' positive and punitive parenting practices. We used information from two survey rounds. Of the 2704 SEED OK participants in the baseline survey, 2259 remained as main caregivers of SEED OK children and completed the follow-up survey in spring 2011 (84% response rate; 1149 in the treatment group, 1110 in the control group). Because the study only included 19 non-Hispanic Asian participants, we excluded them from analyses. We also removed 12 participants for whom values were missing on parenting indicators or demographic characteristics listed in Table 1. The final analytic sample included 2228 primary caregivers: 1130 in the treatment group and 1098 in the control group.

Outcome and independent variables

The outcome variable, parenting practices, was measured in the follow-up survey by six questions from the Alabama Parenting Questionnaire-Preschool Revision, three items for

Table 1. Demographic characteristics and parenting practices of SEED OK participants (*N* = 2228).

Characteristic	Control (*n* = 1098)	Treatment (*n* = 1130)
Child's characteristics		
Male (%)	52.4	53.3
Race (%)		
White	66.4	66.3
African American	9.0	9.1
American Indian	11.6	11.6
Hispanic	13.1	13.1
Mother's characteristics		
Age, *M* (*SD*), by year	25.9 (5.6)	25.8 (5.6)
Education (%)		
Below high school	21.7	20.7
High school	33.4	32.6
Some college	25.5	25.6
4-year college or above	19.4	21.1
Marital status (% married)	62.1	61.0
Household characteristics		
Number of children (%)		
1	34.0	31.7
2	35.9	35.5
3 or more	29.1	31.1
Missing	1.0	1.7
Homeownership (% yes)	43.9	43.3
Received welfare benefits (% yes)	40.1	41.8
Income-to-needs ratio (%)		
<200%	65.6	65.0
200–400%	18.7	18.7
>400%	13.2	12.5
Missing	2.6	4.3
Parenting practices in the follow-up survey		
Praising children, *M* (*SD*), by occurrence	14.7 (13.3)	14.9 (13.6)
Playing with children, *M* (*SD*), by occurrence	8.7 (9.7)	9.0 (9.7)
Explaining to children *M* (*SD*), by occurrence	9.7 (10.6)	9.5 (11.1)
Punishing more, *M* (*SD*), by occurrence[†]	.5 (2.1)	.4 (1.0)
% of zero frequency	81.1	81.5
Spanking children, *M* (*SD*), by occurrence	.7 (1.5)	.6 (1.3)
% of zero frequency	66.3	68.8
Screaming at children, *M* (*SD*), by occurrence [†]	1.6 (3.3)	1.3 (2.7)
% of zero frequency	50.5	51.7

SEED OK = SEED for Oklahoma Kids; 'zero frequency' refers to the frequency with which 0 is assigned as the value for the associated variable. [†]*p* < .10.

positive parenting and another three for punitive parenting (APQ-PR; Clerkin, Halperin, Marks, & Policaro, 2007; Shelton, Frick, & Wootton, 1996). The positive parenting items reported the frequencies of playing a game, praising the child, and calmly explaining the wrong behaviour of the child in a three-day period. The punitive parenting items had frequencies on severe punishment, spanking and screaming at the child in the same period of the time. The treatment status of participants served as the study's independent measure (1 = *treatment group*; 0 = *control group*).

Control variables

The study used multiple demographic and socioeconomic characteristics as control variables. Measured characteristics of the children included gender (1 = *male*; 0 = *female*) and race (non-Hispanic White, non-Hispanic African American, non-Hispanic American Indian, and Hispanic). Measured characteristics of the mothers included age (in years), education (below high school diploma, high school diploma or general equivalency diploma, some college, and 4-year college or above), and marital status (1 = *married*; 0 = *not married*). Several household characteristics also served as control variables. We used four categories to assess the number of children in participants' households: one child, two children, three or more children, and missing value. Nearly 40 mothers did not report this information in the baseline survey. To construct the homeownership variable, we assigned a value of 1 to the variable for homeowners and 0 to the variable for others. To examine welfare programme participation, we assigned a value of 1 to the variable for mothers whose households received Temporary Assistance for Needy Families, food stamps, Supplemental Security Income, or Social Security Disability Insurance benefits in the 12 months prior to the baseline survey. We assigned a value of 0 to the variable for other participants. To create the household income-to-needs ratio, we divided self-reported pretax income in the 12 months before the baseline survey by the appropriate federal poverty guideline for 2007 (Annual Update of the HHS Poverty Guidelines, 2007). To address the missing values in the household income variable (105 mothers reported no value), we assigned sample members to four groups based on the value of their household income-to-needs ratio: <200%, 200%–400%, >400% and missing values.

Statistical analyses

All analyses use structural equation modelling (SEM) in the statistical programme Mplus; we used the estimator of maximum likelihood with robust standard errors for model testing (Muthén & Muthén, 2012). As Figure 3 shows, the SEM analysis had two parts. The first is a measurement model (indicated by solid lines) analysing the relationship between each APQ-PR indicator and the relevant latent variable: positive parenting or punitive parenting. The second is a structural model (indicated by dashed lines) estimating the effect of SEED OK treatment on the latent parenting-practice variables. Analyses were weighted to address self-selection into the SEED OK experiment and sample attrition in the follow-up survey (Schreiner, 2012).

We began the analyses for this study by conducting CFA with data collected by means of the six APQ-PR indicators (i.e. the measurement model). This analysis produced the latent parenting-practice variables: positive parenting and punitive parenting (Kline, 2011). Because they measured the frequency of different parenting behaviours, the six APQ-PR indicators are essentially count variables. As we discuss in the Results section, there is no skew in the distribution of the three indicators on positive parenting. We defined them as continuous variables and used the linear regression to explain the relationship of each to the latent positive-parenting variable. However, the distributions of the punitive indicators were highly skewed. A value of 0 was assigned to the punitive parenting variable for most participants. We thus defined them as count variables and used the zero-inflated Poisson regression to explain each punitive indicator's relationship with the latent punitive-parenting variable (Muthén & Muthén, 2012). To evaluate whether the measurement model fit the data, we compared

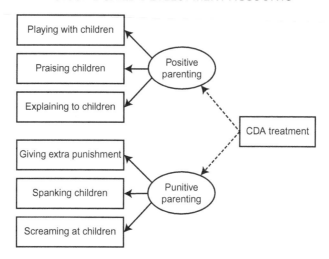

Figure 3. SEM analysis of SEED OK's impacts on positive and punitive parenting.

results from our analysis with estimates from another CFA model that defined all six indicators as continuous variables.

In the second phase of our analyses, we regressed the two latent variables (positive parenting and punitive parenting) on participants' treatment status to assess treatment effects. We did not control for demographic and socioeconomic characteristics in Model 1, and added these control variables in Model 2.

In addition to main the SEM analyses discussed above, we ran two sensitivity tests to examine the robustness of results. The first defined all six APQ-PR indicators as continuous variables in the measurement model, and the second defined all six indicators as count variables in that model. Results from the sensitivity tests were consistent with those from main analyses.

Results

Baseline characteristics

Table 1 presents the baseline characteristics of SEED OK mothers, children, and households. The treatment and control groups did not differ significantly in these characteristics. Table 1 also reports descriptive statistics on the six APR-PR indicators measured at the follow-up survey and presents these by participants' treatment status. On two indicators, the mean scores of treatment mothers were higher than those of control mothers: playing with children (9.0 vs. 8.7) and praising children (14.9 vs. 14.7); however, the score was lower for treatment mothers than for control mothers on the indicator of explaining wrong behaviour to children (9.5 vs. 9.7). The treatment and control groups did not differ significantly on these three indicators. Compared with counterparts in the control group, treatment mothers scored lower on all three punitive indicators: punishing more severely than usual (.4 vs. .5), spanking children (.6 vs. .7), and screaming at children (1.3 vs. 1.6). On the indicators of punishment severity and screaming, the mean treatment–control differences had p-values smaller than .10.

Parenting practices and CFA

The first column of Table 2 (CFA with count variables) lists results of the CFA measurement model in which the three punitive indicators were defined as count variables. We report both factor loadings and model fit information. Because the CFA included count variables, we present nonstandardised factor loadings. The chi-square test for count variables produced a nonsignficiant result (χ = 654.24; df = 986; and p = 1.00), which suggests that the model was an acceptable fit for count outcomes.

However, several commonly used fit indices (e.g. the root mean square error of approximation, the Tucker Lewis index, the comparative fit index, the standardised root mean square residual) are not suitable for the CFA with count variables. For the purposes of comparison, the second column in Table 2 (CFA with continuous variables) reports standardised factor loadings and model fit indices for the CFA measurement model in which all six parenting indicators were defined as continuous variables. Except for Tucker Lewis index, which was less than .90, the values of standardised factor loadings and model fit indices mentioned above suggest that this comparison CFA model had a reasonable fit to the data. More importantly, comparative model fit indices (Akaike information criterion, Bayesian information criterion and sample-size-adjusted Bayesian information criterion) in the first column were all greater than those in the second column, and the difference indicated that the CFA model with count variables fit the data better than the model reported in the second column.

Impacts of SEED OK on parenting practices

Table 3 reports main results from an analysis regressing the positive- and punitive-parenting variables on participants' treatment status. Full results can be requested from the authors. Because the measurement scales of latent variables were not defined, we

Table 2. Model fit of CFA analyses (N = 2228).

Factor loading and model fit	CFA with count variables	CFA with continuous variables
Factor loading for positive parenting		
Praising children	1.00	0.75
Playing with children	0.67	0.72
Explaining to children	0.71	0.67
Factor loading for punitive parenting		
Punishing more	1.00	0.52
Spanking children	0.74	0.66
Screaming at children	0.85	0.60
Correlation between two factors	0.30	0.31
Model fit		
χ test for count variables (df)	654.24 (986)	
AIC	64,054.94	76,039.99
BIC	64,163.41	76,148.46
Sample-size adjusted BIC	64,103.04	76,088.09
RMSEA [90% CI]		.04
		[.03, .06]
CFI		.91
TLI		.84
SRMR		.04

CFA = confirmatory factor analysis; df = degrees of freedom; AIC = Akaike information criterion; BIC = Bayesian information criterion; CI = confidence interval; RMSEA = root mean square error of approximation; CFI = comparative fit index; TLI = Tucker Lewis index; SRMR = standardised root mean square residual.

Table 3. Impacts of SEED OK on parenting practices (N = 2228).

Variables	Model 1		Model 2	
	Punitive parenting	Positive parenting	Punitive parenting	Positive parenting
Main analysis: Punitive parenting indicators defined as count variables				
Treatment group	−.06*	.00	−.12*	.01
	(0.3)	(.03)	(.06)	(.05)
Sensitivity Test 1: All parenting indicators defined as continuous variables				
Treatment group	−.05[†]	.00	−.09[†]	.01
	(0.3)	(.03)	(.05)	(.05)
Sensitivity Test 2: All parenting indicators defined as count variables				
Treatment group	−.06*	−.00	−.12*	−.01
	(0.3)	(.02)	(.06)	(.05)

SEED OK = SEED for Oklahoma Kids. Results are standardised, and standard errors are shown in parentheses.
[†]$p < .10$.
*$p < .05$.

standardised positive parenting and punitive parenting so that they had a mean of 0 and a standard deviation of 1 (Kline, 2011). In the main analyses, Model 1 did not control for demographic and socioeconomic characteristics. The standardised regression coefficient showed that the treatment and control groups did not differ significantly on the mean value of the positive-parenting variable ($B = .00$). However, the mean value of the punitive-parenting variables for treatment mothers was .06 standard deviations smaller than that for control mothers ($B = −.06$; $p < .05$). Model 2 adjusted for control variables listed in Table 1, and the results indicated that the mean value of the punitive-parenting variable was .12 standard deviations smaller for treatment mothers than for control mothers. Model 2 explained about 5.3% of the variance on the latent punitive-parenting variable. If estimated without the treatment status variable, Model 2 explained only 4.9% of the variance on punitive parenting. That is, the R-squared change caused by the SEED OK intervention was .4%.

Discussion

The results indicated that punitive parenting practices, measured in the follow-up survey, were significantly less frequent among treatment mothers than among control mothers but that the two groups did not differ significantly on positive parenting practices. The SEED OK intervention appears to have reduced the frequency of punitive-parenting behaviours among treatment mothers. This evidence partially supports the hypothesis that CDAs affect parenting practices.

The size of SEED OK's effect on punitive parenting (.12, Table 3) seems modest. One strategy for interpreting the effect size is to compare it with the parenting effects of some early childhood programmes. For example, one project found that participation in the Head Start programme reduced punitive parenting (indicated by the parent's use of spanking in the week prior to survey) at the end of the Head Start year, with an effect size of .14. The study also found that, by the end of the kindergarten year, participation reduced the parent's use of time out as a tool for disciplining his or her child, and the effect size was .13 (U.S. Department of Health and Human Services, 2010). Also, Love et al. (2005) evaluated the Early Head Start programme's effects on parenting, finding that it reduced the frequency with which parents spanked their children in the week prior to assessment. The estimated effect size was less than .30.

Taking all of this previous research into consideration, the effect size of reduction in punitive parenting practices in SEED OK can be described as modest yet meaningful. It is important to note that the SEED OK intervention to build financial assets is also a less direct approach than those taken by parenting and early-childhood programmes. And the financial investment in SEED OK (a maximum of $2100; most treatment mothers received only $1000) was comparatively small. In addition, SEED OK treatment families retained this investment themselves, that is, the money was not 'spent' but rather transferred. In this sense, the 'expense' of SEED OK can be described as near zero. Given very low costs and indirect effect, SEED OK's modest yet meaningful impact on punitive parenting is perhaps especially noteworthy.

This experiment with CDAs did not examine the process by which the SEED OK intervention affected parenting practices. The qualitative data from 60 SEED OK mothers suggested that SEED OK motivated mothers, especially those with disadvantaged backgrounds, 'to see their children as college bound' and to increase support for children's education in the precollege years (Gray, Clancy, Sherraden, Wagner, & Miller-Cribbs, 2012, p. 76). Improvements in parenting practices and reductions in punitive parenting can be considered forms of such support.

Previous research has indicated that the SEED OK intervention raised parents' educational expectations, reduced their depressive symptoms and improved children's social–emotional development (Huang et al., 2014, Huang et al., 2014; Kim et al., 2015). The current study's finding on parenting practices is consistent with those treatment effects.

Study limitations should also be noted. First, although the psychometric features of the APQ-PR have been tested, this study used six APQ-PR questions whose validity and reliability have not been established. A related issue is that parenting style, another important aspect of parenting, was not measured in the SEED OK follow-up survey. Future research should use a fuller measure of parenting to evaluate the impact of CDAs, and that measure should examine parenting styles. Second, treatment mothers might have intentionally misreported parenting practices to make their parenting seem more favourable than it actually was. The intervention's financial incentives and several other factors may have motivated this sort of embellishment. However, nonsignificance of the treatment–control difference in positive parenting implied that the estimate were not likely to suffer from the Hawthorne effect. Otherwise, we should have found that the SEED OK intervention had positive impacts on positive parenting as well. Finally, the participation rate in the research was low (37%). Another 17% of participants were lost from the analysis due to sample attrition in the follow-up survey. Treatment and control groups were well balanced in the final analytic sample based on observable characteristics, but the issues above leave open the possibility of selection bias, and therefore external validity.

Findings from this study add to the mounting evidence that CDAs, an economic intervention designed to build assets for children, have favourable effects on child development and parenting behaviours. In this study, we found that the intervention reduced punitive parenting. It is noteworthy that the SEED OK intervention differed from traditional parenting interventions (e.g. home visits) in that the CDAs did not include information on parenting or training on parenting skills. Improving parenting skills is considered a key strategy to reduce and prevent children's behaviour problems and to promote overall child well-being. Policymakers might consider combining CDAs with other child development initiatives, including parenting education. In this way, a CDA might better function as an additional tool to support child development.

Findings from the present study and previous SEED OK research suggest that the universal, automatic, and progressive CDA in the SEED OK experiment has efficiently achieved the goal of full-population participation, and also improved families' financial and nonfinancial outcomes. These are the critical design features of large-scale CDAs, and should be applied to the CDA development and implementation in the global context.

Acknowledgments

Support for the SEED for Oklahoma Kids experiment comes from the Ford Foundation and Charles Stewart Mott Foundation. We especially value our partnership with the State of Oklahoma: Ken Miller, State Treasurer; Scott Meacham, former State Treasurer; Tim Allen, Deputy Treasurer for Communications and Program Administration; and James Wilbanks, former Director of Revenue and Fiscal Policy. We appreciate the contributions of staff at RTI International, especially those of Ellen Marks and Bryan Rhodes. The Oklahoma 529 College Savings Plan Program Manager, TIAA-CREF, has also been a valuable partner. We are grateful to Mark Schreiner, Sandy Beverly, and Youngmi Kim for their careful review and insightful comments; to Mark Schreiner and Nora Wikoff for their assistance in managing the survey data; to Chris Leiker and John Gabbert for providing editorial assistance; and to staff on the SEED OK team over several years.

Disclosure statement

No potential conflict of interest was reported by the authors.

Funding

This work is supported by the Ford Foundation and Charles Stewart Mott Foundation.

References

Annual Update of the HHS Poverty Guidelines, 72 Fed. Reg. 3147 (notice issued January 24, 2007).

Aunola, K., & Nurmi, J.-E. (2005). The role of parenting styles in children's problem behavior. *Child Development, 76*(6), 1144–1159.

Belsky, J., & Jaffee, S. R. (2006). The multiple determinants of parenting. In D. Cicchetti & D. J. Cohen (Eds.), *Developmental psychopathology: Vol. 3. Risk, disorder, and adaptation* (2nd ed., pp. 38–85). New York, NY: Wiley.

Beverly, S. G., Kim, Y., Sherraden, M., Nam, Y., & Clancy, M. (2015). Can child development accounts be inclusive? Early evidence from a statewide experiment. *Children and Youth Services Review, 53*, 92–104.

Capaldi, D. M., Chamberlain, P., & Patterson, G. R. (1997). Ineffective discipline and conduct problems in males: Association, late adolescent outcomes, and prevention. *Aggression and Violent Behavior, 2*, 343–353.

Chaffin, M., & Friedrich, B. (2004). Evidence-based treatments in child abuse and neglect. *Children and Youth Service Review, 26*(11), 1097–1113.

Clancy, M., Beverly, S., Sherraden, M., & Huang, J. (2016). Testing universal child development accounts: Financial effects in a large social experiment. *Social Service Review, 90*(4), 683–708.

Clancy, M., & Sherraden, M. (2014). *Automatic deposits for all at birth: Maine's Harold Alfond college challenge* (CSD Policy Report 14-05). St. Louis, MO: Washington University, Center for Social Development.

Clerkin, S. M., Halperin, J. M., Marks, D. J., & Policaro, K. L. (2007). Psychometric properties of the Alabama parenting questionnaire–Preschool revision. *Journal of Clinical Child & Adolescent Psychology, 36*(1), 19–28.

Darling, N., & Steinberg, L. (1993). Parenting style as context: An integrative model. *Psychological Bulletin, 113*(3), 487–496.

Elder, G. H., Jr., Eccles, J. S., Ardelt, M., & Lord, S. (1995). Inner-city parents under economic pressure: Perspectives on the stratgies of parenting. *Journal of Marriage and the Family, 57*(3), 771–784.

Gershoff, E. T. (2002). Corporal punishment by parents and associated child behaviors and experiences: A meta-analytic and theoretical review. *Psychological Bulletin, 128*(4), 539–579.

Gray, K., Clancy, M., Sherraden, M. S., Wagner, K., & Miller-Cribbs, J. (2012). *Interviews with mothers of young children in the SEED for Oklahoma Kids college savings experiment* (CSD Research Report No. 12-53). St. Louis, MO: Washington University, Center for Social Development. Retrieved from http://csd.wustl.edu/Publications/Documents/RP12-53.pdf

Huang, J., Sherraden, M., Kim, Y., & Clancy, M. (2014). Effects of child development accounts on early social-emotional development: An experimental test. *JAMA pediatrics, 168*(3), 265–271.

Huang, J., Sherraden, M., & Purnell, J. Q. (2014). Impacts of child development accounts on maternal depressive symptoms: Evidence from a randomized statewide policy experiment. *Social Science & Medicine, 112*, 30–38.

Kim, Y., Sherraden, M., Huang, J., & Clancy, M. (2015). Child development accounts and parental educational expectations for young children: Early evidence from a statewide social experiment. *Social Service Review, 89*(1), 99–137.

King, J. (2014, February 10). Senator Ron Wyden wants children's savings accounts [Web log post]. Retrieved from http://assets.newamerica.net/blogposts/2014/senator_ron_wyden_wants_childrens_savings_accounts-103297

Kline, R. B. (2011). *Principles and practice of structural equation modeling* (3rd ed.). New York, NY: Guilford.

Linver, M. R., Brooks-Gunn, J., & Kohen, D. E. (2002). Family processes as pathways from income to young children's development. *Developmental Psychology, 38*(5), 719–734.

Love, J. M., Kisker, E. E., Ross, C., Raikes, H., Constantine, J., Boller, K., . . . Vogel, C. (2005). The effectiveness of early head start for 3-year-old children and their parents: Lessons for policy and programs. *Developmental Psychology, 41*(6), 885–901.

MacLeod, J., & Nelson, G. (2000). Programs for the promotion of family wellness and the prevention of child maltreatment: A meta-analytic review. *Child Abuse & Neglect, 24*(9), 1127–1149.

Meyer, J., Masa, R. D., & Zimmerman, J. M. (2010). Overview of child development accounts in developing countries. *Children and Youth Services Review, 32*(11), 1561–1569.

Muthén, L. K., & Muthén, B. O. (2012). *Mplus. The comprehensive modelling program for applied researchers: User's guide* (7th ed.). Los Angeles, CA: Muthén & Muthén.

Nam, Y., Kim, Y., Clancy, M., Zager, R., & Sherraden, M. (2013). Do child development accounts promote account holding, saving, and asset accumulation for children's future? Evidence from a statewide randomized experiment. *Journal of Policy Analysis and Management, 32*(1), 6–33.

Nam, Y., Wikoff, N., & Sherraden, M. (2014). Economic intervention and parenting: A randomized experiment of a statewide child development account program. *Research on Social Work Practice, 26*(4), 339–349.

New America Foundation. (2013). The ASPIRE act of 2013: The america saving for personal investment, retirement, and education act (Section-by-section of the proposed legislation). Retrieved from http://assets.newamerica.net/sites/newamerica.net/files/program_pages/attach ments/ASPIRE%202013%20Section%20by%20Section.pdf

Patterson, G. R. (2002). The early development of coercive family process. In J. B. Reid, G. R. Patterson, & J. Snyder (Eds.), *Antisocial behavior in children and adolescents: A developmental analysis and model for intervention* (pp. 25–44). Washington, DC: American Psychological Association.

Schreiner, M. (2012). *Meta-data for SEED for Oklahoma Kids: Two survey waves and OSCP administrative data through 2011Q4* (Report). St. Louis, MO: Washington University, Center for Social Development.

Segal, L., Opie, R. S., & Dalziel, K. (2012). Theory! The missing link in understanding the performance of neonate/infant home-visiting programs to prevent child maltreatment: A systematic review. *Milbank Quarterly, 90*(1), 47–106.

Shelton, K. K., Frick, P. J., & Wootton, J. (1996). Assessment of parenting practices in families of elementary school-age children. *Journal of Clinical Child Psychology, 25*(3), 317–329.

Sherraden, M. (1991). *Assets and the poor: A new American welfare policy.* Armonk, NY: M. E. Sharpe.

Sherraden, M., Clancy, C., Nam, Y., Huang, J., Kim, Y., Beverly, S., ... Purnell, J. Q. (2015). Universal accounts at birth: Building knowledge to inform policy. *Journal of the Society for Social Work and Research, 6*(4), 541–564.

Shonkoff, J. P., & Phillips, D. A. (Eds.). (2000). *From neurons to neighborhoods: The science of early childhood development.* Washington, DC: National Academies Press.

Thomlison, B. (2004). Child maltreatment: A risk and protective factor perspective. In M. W. Fraser (Ed.), *Risk and resilience in childhood: An ecological perspective* (2nd ed., pp. 89–132). Washington DC: NASW Press.

U.S. Department of Health and Human Services, Administration for Children and Families, Office of Planning, Research and Evaluation. (2010). Head start impact study: Final report. Retrieved from http://www.acf.hhs.gov/sites/default/files/opre/hs_impact_study_final.pdf

U.S. Department of the Treasury. (2009 September 9). *An analysis of section 529 college savings and prepaid tuition plans: A report prepared by the department of treasury for the white house task force on middle class working families* (Report). Retrieved from http://www.treasury.gov/ resource-center/economic-policy/Documents/09092009TreasuryReportSection529.pdf

Verhoeven, M., Junger, M., Van Aken, C., Deković, M., & Van Aken, M. A. (2007). Parenting during toddlerhood: Contributions of parental, contextual, and child characteristics. *Journal of Family Issues, 28*(12), 1663–1691.

Zhan, M., & Sherraden, M. (2003). Assets, expectations, and children's educational achievement in female-headed households. *Social Service Review, 77*(2), 191–211.

Policy innovation and policy realisation: the example of children future education and development accounts in Taiwan

Li-Chen Cheng

ABSTRACT

The Children Future Education and the Development Accounts (CFEDAs) are the first anti-poverty policy in Taiwan developed to provide incentives for the poor to accumulate assets for their future. Using CFEDAs as an example, this article analyses the process of developing and implementing an asset-based policy. It begins with an introduction to the policy structure. It then reviews the history of how the innovative idea of building assets for the poor became a policy proposal before presenting the convergence of three policy streams driving the prioritisation of CFEDAS in Taiwan's policy agenda. It concludes with challenges facing the policy implementation.

Introduction

Children are the future of society. Investing in their education is a core value in Asian culture. However, many children live in poverty as a result of family economic hardship, with many others being forced from their homes because of their family's inability to support their regular living. The child poverty rate in Taiwan fluctuated between 5% and 9%, centring on the rate of 7%, in the past two decades (Lee & Wang, 2011). Moreover, children aged younger than 18 years account for 30%–40% of the low-income population receiving public assistance (Lee & Wang, 2011). Such poverty hinders the normal development of children; for example, they face short- and long-term consequences on their psychosocial development and have limited life chances in adulthood (Duncan & Brooks-Gunn, 1997; Leu, Chen, & Chen, 2016).

Public concern over child poverty raised in Taiwan. However, child and adult poverty are significantly interrelated. Adult poverty can be traced back to childhood: poor investment in human capital during early developmental age, a lack of asset-building opportunities and low involvement in labour markets in childhood have lifelong effects that extend into adulthood (Bradbury, 2003).

Based on the principle of income-based financial transfers, Taiwan's public assistance system traditionally fills the income gap between household income and the poverty line to maintain the basic living standards of the poor (Sun, 1995). Moreover, Taiwan lifted employment barriers for the working poor as a means to strengthen their economic sufficiency. However, Taiwan's dramatic economic recession in 1999 led to a sharp increase in working individuals applying for public assistance; therefore, welfare reform was called for to address the ineffective anti-poverty strategy (Cheng, 2000).

To address this issue, President Tsai, Ing-wen proposed a policy, the Children Future Education and the Development Accounts (CFEDAs), to Taiwan's Legislative Yuan on 1 December 2017. Shortly thereafter, the Legislative Yuan passed the CFEDA policy proposal with a bi-partisan support, and President Tsai, Ing-wen signed the bill into law on 6 June 2018.

Drawing heavily from Sherraden's asset-based welfare theory (Sherraden, 1991), CFEDAs are the first anti-poverty policy in Taiwan developed to provide incentives for the poor to build assets for their future, gain access to financial information and make investments in a planned way. Through long-term asset building and matched savings, CFEDAs are designed to help Taiwan's poor and fostered children escape economic hardship, increase their chances of getting higher education and develop careers later in adulthood.

This article describes the policy structure of CFEDAs, reviews the history of how the innovative idea of building assets for the poor became a policy proposal and presents three policy streams driving the prioritisation of CFEDAs in Taiwan's policy agenda. It concludes with future challenges facing the implementation of CFEDAs.

Policy structure of the CFEDAs

'Investing in children is investing in our future' is the slogan for CFEDAs. The policy invests in children by offering them matched saving accounts over an 18-year period. This section details the policy structure of the CFEDAs by discussing the eligible population, account features and policy design

Eligible population

Taiwanese children born after 1 January 2016 from poor families or fostered children who are under government custody are eligible for CFEDA benefits. Taiwan conducts a means-test process to deem families poor and enlist them as low income in the welfare register. Newborn children from poor families who enlist in the welfare register are eligible to open a CFEDA. They could receive publicly subsidised matched savings in their CFEDA every year until they reach the age of 18. If the family moves out of poverty before their children reach the age of 18, they are able to continue depositing money into their CFEDA and/or earn annual saving interests, without matched savings temporarily (unless they lapse back into poverty and reenlist in the welfare register). Children fostered out-of-home for over 2 years with custodianship granted to the government are also eligible. According to the Ministry of Health and Welfare (2018), more than 3,000 children are placed in foster homes or residential programs every year. Among them, only about 600–700 are eligible for CFEDAs.

As of this writing (August, 2018), there are 12,624 children eligible to participate in the CFEDA program (Li, Pi-Yi, Director of the Ministry of Health and Welfare, personal communication, August 2, 2018). The government projects a 30% enrolment rate in CFEDAs for the first year. This figure is based on the response rate to a question on the 2013 Survey on Middle and Low Income Families that asked about income balance after public transfer: 28.7 % of the interviewees indicated having well-balanced family income. As of August, 2018, Director Li indicated in the conversation that 4,587 eligible children have enrolled and 3,944 have opened accounts, with about a 36% enrolment rate for eligible children enrolling and 31% opening accounts. Therefore, the CFEDA policy has achieved its first year enrolment projection. In the future, more strategies are needed to increase enrolment and include more eligible children.

Account features

Participating children could receive an initial deposit of as much as NT$10,000 (approximately US$335) into their CFEDA. Participants' parents or legal guardians could choose between three monthly saving levels of NT$500 (approximately US$17), NT$1,000, (approximately US$33) and NT$1,250 (approximately US$42). The government would match these deposit levels at a 1:1 ratio with a maximum of NT $15,000 (approximately US$500) per year, adding up to a maximum of NT$30,000 (approximately US$1,000) assets per year for each participant. If they do not drop out, each participant is expected to have a maximum of NT$ 540,000 (approximately US $18,000) by the time they reach the age of 18. Participants' parents or legal guardians receive a bank statement every 6 months that detail the total amount of their deposits and matched savings. Withdrawals are restricted to emergencies, such as death of a child, serious health problems and other event of force majeure.

When CFEDAs are mature, the participants are encouraged to use the accumulated assets to pay for higher education, occupational training or business start-up fund; however, it is not mandated. Every participant needs to submit an application to indicate the purpose of the expenditure using funds from his or her CFEDA. If the specific plan for the money is not specified, withdrawal of the matched fund may be denied. To discourage participants from recklessly spending assets, the Ministry of Health and Welfare provides financial education to participants and their parents on how to invest savings in financial institutions, social service agencies and schools in an intentional way. If necessary, personal counselling is available to participants who need assistance making plans for using their savings. Financial institutions can also provide information for participants to transfer their saving to other financial products.

Design

Suggested by Beverly and Sherraden (1999), an individual's willingness to save could facilitate his or her conscious decision to postpone consumption and to save more in a contractual savings scheme. Therefore, to encourage savings, participation in CFEDAs is designed to be voluntary. To motivate children from low-income families to participate, the CFEDAs are designed to include the assistance of family social workers. Participants who have not yet enrolled or could not make regular deposit can be referred to a home-visiting program. The needy welfare resources or in-kind services mitigate possible economic crises and remove barriers to making deposits.

To reinforce participants and their parents' saving behaviour and increase their financial capability, the Ministry of Health and Welfare is currently collaborating with the Financial Social Worker Center of Fu-Jen University to develop financial education modules and materials. The Center has developed several financial courses, such as

'My Financial Condition', 'Cash Flow and Book Keeping', 'My Dream of Spending Map', 'Strategies for Smart Spending', 'Can I Increase My Income?' and 'Foster Better Saving Behaviours'. The courses will train social workers of home-visiting programs and the first-year CFEDAs enrollers' parents to assess the efficacy of the modules or materials in increasing financial literacy and changing saving behaviours.

The CFEDAs are also designed to include three primary incentives for participating families. First, assets held in CFEDAs are exempt from the means-tested calculation that imposes a strict eligibility level for low-income benefits in Taiwan. Therefore, families saving in CFEDAs need not worry about losing their welfare benefits. Second, CFEDAs are designed to allow private donors to contribute to or sponsor accounts as supplementary deposits. However, the matched savings the government provides applies only to the saving amount of each of three saving levels, and not the supplementary deposits. Third, CFEDAs are designed so that interest accrues regularly from the Bank of Taiwan – a publicly owned bank – on deposits into the accounts. Every participant receives an account statement every 6 months as a reminder of their deposit level.

From policy innovation towards policy realisation

According to Sherraden (2001), a new policy cannot be initiated on its own. Instead, policy formulation is an incremental process that builds momentum over time. The contextual forces, mainly political and socio-economic transformations, provide opportunities for new concepts and policy innovation to take place. This holds true in the case of Taiwan. This section discusses the political history of modern Taiwan and how it has affected its socio-economic transformation and policy landscape.

Ending martial law and beginning democracy

Politically, in 1988, the Nationalist government abolished martial law, putting an end to an authoritarian regime of centralised control. As a result, local governments and civil groups were given more power to pursue their best interests. In 1994, for the first time in modern history, Taipei citizens elected the mayor rather than someone being appointed by the central government. The newfound political autonomy created competing political parties and, thus, a strong driving force for policy innovation.

During the second mayoral elections of 1997, a new approach to public assistance based on asset accumulation was initiated. The idea of matched savings for the poor had bipartisan support from both the incumbent mayor and the opponent because its core values of ownership were tied closely with Chinese values on savings and assets (Chang, 1993). In 2000, the Taipei City Government launched the 3-year Taipei Family Development Accounts (TFDAs) project to assist low-income working households to accumulate major assets in life. The launch of TFDAs marked the first anti-poverty initiative that incentivises low-income families to save and accumulate assets to achieve economic self-sufficiency (Cheng, 2003).

Recession and the road to recovery

Taiwan has been referred to as one of 'the four tigers' in East Asia, exemplifying the story of fast-growing economies in the region during the 1980s (Dahlman & Sanaikone, 1997). However, the global economic recession since the mid-1990s has slowed Taiwan's rapid and sustained economic growth (Haggard, 2001; Krongkaew, 2002), which witnessed a sharp decline in asset values, falling real wages and rising unemployment rates (Haggard, 2001; Lee, 2002). Therefore, there is urgent need for new social contracts to reduce the high social costs of growing economic inequality, especially the asset disparity between the rich and the poor (Cheng, 2003). Asset-building policies for the poor, such as TFDAs and CFEDAs, provide a solution to address the inequality issue.

Asset policy diffusion and social change

According to Mintrom (2000), the actions of policy experts who promote policy ideas raise the probability of legislative consideration and approval of policy innovations. In this *policy diffusion* process, policy experts spot problems, promote innovative approaches to problem-solving and shaping policy debates and work to build networked coalitions to support policy innovation (Mintrom, 2000). Developing innovation should be followed by implementing innovation (McDaniel, 2000).

In the case of Taiwan, policy diffusion took place in the form of building assets for the poor (Zou et al., 2013). Informed by the Taipei City Government implementation of TFDAs, a number of local governments in Taiwan have launched their own asset-based policies and programs. With the diffusion trajectory from north to south and urban to rural, the innovative idea and demonstration stories are becoming common anti-poverty measures (Zou et al., 2013). After the establishment of TFDAs, academic scholars and program managers spent a significant amount of time networking in and around schools and local governments. Academic scholars interfaced at both academic and policy fields, shaping the debates of innovative policy ideas at academic conferences and in classrooms, while learning of the rich experiences from the program implementation (Zou et al., 2013). Program managers presented the prototype design of small-scale asset-building programs to potential interest groups. These efforts led to growing networks and coalitions of policymakers and welfare scholars. It manifested in what Mintrom (2000) described as the crucial roles that networked policy experts play in initiating dynamic policy change, articulating policy innovation onto government agenda, and energising the diffusion process.

Taiwan's 2016 presidential campaign created another opportunity for social change. During the previous 8 years, the public was largely dissatisfied with President, Ma, Ying-jeou's administration's imbalanced and pro-big-business policies. In his analysis, Yang (2015) presented that real wages contracted by 2.6 % from 2001 to 2014, while real GDP increased by 71 % over the same period. The link between real wage growth and GDP growth in Taiwan dramatically decreased, revealing how corporate earnings were not trickling down to their employees. Consequently, young people aged between 15 and 24 suffered high unemployment, with rates at 8% in 2000 and increasing to 13.17% in 2014. The nation's uneven distribution of wealth, sluggish wage increase and high unemployment became the most controversial issues in the presidential debates (Yang, 2015).

A changing society

At the same time, Taiwanese society experienced a sharp demographic change. It was reported (National Development Council, 2014) that people older than 65 accounted for 7% of the whole population since 1993, and it is estimated to reach 14% by 2018 and

24.1% in 2030. Moreover, the average number of children that would be born to a woman over her lifetime (the total fertility rate) was 2.15 in 1983, and sharply dropped to the rate of 1.06 in 2015. If this trend continues, Taiwan's aging society would soon reach the levels of European nations introducing a number of challenges to family sustainability and the government's ability to support the aging population. During the presidential debates in 2015, the two candidates were requested to address imbalanced demographic development. In the debate, the issues of developing a long-term care system for the elderly and a friendly childcare system to boost the birth rate were extensively and heatedly discussed. Then candidate Tsai especially discussed her duty to develop a social safety net for the children by investing in their future.

The asset-building coalition

Before her eventual election in 2016, then candidate Tsai invited several welfare scholars as consultants to draft social welfare policies included in her campaign manifestation. As mentioned above, during policy innovation and diffusion process of asset-based programs, an increasingly networked coalition of policymakers, program managers and welfare scholars who favoured building assets for the poor was formed. In consultation meetings with Tsai's administration, this coalition proposed a policy of poverty reduction based on matched savings for children. Tsai, Ing-wen quickly adopted the idea and included it in her implementation list of social welfare policies. The government used to have anti-poverty programmes for a two or three year term. But the Accounts will open an account for every eligible child for 18 years. Therefore, the Accounts is a long term policy, instead of a shor-term programme.

Three streams of developing the CFEDAs

According to Kingdon (1986), how certain problems are deemed significant enough to get on a political agenda (whereas others do not) is determined by how a policy agenda is developed. He indicated that an agenda being favoured politically can be the result of three converging streams: (1) the problem stream, (2) the policy stream and (3) the politics stream. First, the problem may be brought to the attention of policymakers through various ways. Second, proposals must meet certain criteria concerning equity, technically feasibility and congruence with society's values. Third, some events must occur to lead the government to take actions or make changes. This section examines how these three streams contributed to the development of the CFEDAs policy proposal in Taiwan.

The problem stream

Taiwan realising the policy innovation of building assets for the poor demonstrates a convergence of several driving forces to make the CFEDAs the priority of the Tsai administration's policy agenda. In terms of a problem stream, the issue of child poverty was brought to policymakers' attention by the media and interest groups. According to one study (Lee & Wang, 2011), the child poverty rate (the number of children below poverty line over the total children population) in Taiwan had increased. The rate increased to 8.03% in 1993, before fluctuating between 5% and 9% from 1988 to 2009. But the rates increased again to 7.7% in 2009. In addition to the instability of these figures, research indicated that living in poverty has negative impacts on Taiwanese children's cognitive development process and life chances in the future (Leu et al., 2016). Therefore, this problem stream led policymakers to request the central government to adopt a more effective approach to reducing poverty vulnerability among families with children, such as developing asset-building accounts for poor children.

Most Taiwanese children from low-income families require student loans to pay for their higher education. As a result of the 2000 financial crisis, many students had to drop out of college because they were unable to afford tuition fees (Kuo et al., 2013). To ease the issue, the government began subsidising student loans to low-income families by paying the interest accrued on their loans. According to the statistics of student loans provided by the Ministry of Education (2018), there has been a dramatic increase in the number of student loan borrowers and the total amount of lending during this time period. Between 2000 and 2010, the number of student loan borrowers more than doubled, from 339,291 to 777,305. Accordingly, the amount of interest subsidisation the Central Government had to pay the bank increased dramatically. For example, public expenditure allocates 30 to 40 million NT$ per year to subsidise student loan interests.

The rapid growth in outstanding debt had a profound impact on student borrowers. When the borrowers graduated, they had to begin repaying the loans after 1 year of deferment. The repayment, paired with low pay and high unemployment facing Taiwanese young people, devastated the borrowers' chances of upward mobility. In effect, banks – not students – benefited from student loan policy in Taiwan. The issue raised public demand for a policy that directly invests in students' education, rather than investing in banks.

The policy stream

As the problem stream generated greater public awareness, policymakers noticed and the policy stream followed suit. As a result, investment in children's education is now strongly favoured as a way to promote human capital to escape from poverty in Taiwan. The CFEDAs serve as a suitable policy solution because they emphasise investing in children's education rather than providing welfare benefits. Moreover, this concept fits well with Chinese culture, which values educational investment. From the perspective of policymakers, receiving higher education is an effective path to upward mobility and breaking the intergenerational vicious cycle of poverty. On the other hand, they see encouraging students to borrow loans as a consumption strategy. Because it provides more than 3.2 billion NT$ annually in interest subsidies on student loans, the Taiwanese government also benefits from CFEDAs. Once the CFEDAs mature, the savers could use the assets to pay for their higher education, thus reducing this expenditure.

Sherraden's idea of asset-based welfare theory has been in practice in Taiwan since 2000, and policy diffusion has been ongoing ever since. The networked coalitions are the key actors in policy diffusion: They initiate dynamic policy change, articulate policy innovations onto government agenda and energise the diffusion process. They identify problems, network in the policy arena, shape policy debates and build coalitions to support policy innovations (Mintrom, 2000). Moreover, academic scholars interface at both academic and policy levels, shape the debates of innovative policy ideas at academic conferences and in classrooms and learn rich experiences from the program implementation (McDaniel, 2000). Under this diffusion background, the idea of asset building as an effective anti-poverty strategy has been corroborated. In Taiwan, because policymakers and welfare scholars had been made familiar with the theoretical framework (i.e. the policy stream), CFEDAs policy was proposed and eventually enacted.

Politics stream

Regarding the politics stream, an event increased public attention before the presidential election. In March of 2014, a group of college students started the Sunflower Movement. The students occupied government offices and partially paralysed the political system. The movement's goal was to protest Taiwan's trade agreement with China. With a large number of student demonstrators, it captured the attention of nearly everyone in Taiwan and even the foreign media. Observers conjectured that the basis for the students' dissatisfaction was Taiwan's poorly performing economy, lack of jobs for graduates and opportunities drying up everywhere (except in China). The young people's voices had a keen impact on the presidential election in 2016.

As mentioned above, when a political paradigm shifts, it provides a good opportunity for new social policy to be enacted. The 2016 election of Tsai, Ing-wen represents this idea in action. In casting their votes, young people played a key role in the outcome of the election. Tsai promised to promote social equality and more opportunities for the young people in response to their strong support. Therefore, the CFEDAs policy initiative was launched on 1 June 2017, a bill containing the CFEDAs was sent into the Legislative Yuan for law making at the end of 2017, and it was passed on July, 2018. President Tsai, Ing-wen signed the bill to promulgate laws on June 6. On that day, she proclaimed a victory in investing in children and Taiwan's future.

Challenges ahead

So far, this article has examined the policy structure of the CFEDAs, the accumulating process of policy innovation to policy realisation and the convergence of three policy streams of prioritising CFEDAs in Taiwan's government policy agenda. Despite their early success, CFEDAs will face some challenges ahead in their implementation.

By design, CFEDAs' participation is voluntary. In the first year, CFEDAs reached a 36% enrolment rate for eligible children enrolling with 31% opening accounts, which meets the projected 30% participation rate. Though initial enrolments are promising, additional promoting strategies are necessary to increase the enrolment rate and ensure the long-term success of CFEDAs. According to social workers who visited eligible participants, some were unfamiliar with the enrolling process, lacked information about the policy or were not motivated. Therefore, removing these barriers is necessary to include more eligible participants in future implementation.

Given these barriers, families with eligible children must be encouraged to at least open a CFEDA and make an initial deposit in this early stage of implementation. The government disseminates information regarding the program structure and enrolment procedures to low-income families through the media and other channels. To increase future account enrolment, information about CFEDA incentives should be presented clearly and effectively through home-visiting programs. Along with implementation, more research on parents' motivation, attitudes and aspiration of enrolment is needed to develop more effective enrolment alternatives, such as an automatic enrolment design (with the option to opt out). Therefore, these enrolment alternatives could be amended into the policy in the future.

Another challenge will involve how to reinforce CFEDA holders' saving behaviours in implementation. CFEDAs provide matched savings to each participant. To encourage saving, added incentives will be pertinent in maintaining accountholders' saving habits (Beverly & Sherraden, 1999). Though CFEDAs are designed to include some incentives, such as account savings exempted from means-tested calculation and the ability for private donors to contribute or sponsor accounts, more are necessary. During the planning phase for CFEDAs, several child welfare organisations were invited to provide suggestions for program structure design. They indicated an interest in being community partners to accountholders by making supplementary deposits into their accounts. However, the supplementary nature of the deposits is not regular saving sources. In the future, the policy structure should include such supplementary deposits as primary saving sources to enable eligible children to accelerate accumulating assets.

After participants open accounts and start to save, developing their financial literacy and capability can lead to better economic outcomes (Adams & Beverly, 2013). Therefore, another challenge in ensuring the success of CFEDAs will involve increasing financial education to build such knowledge and skills. The financial education modules being developed by the Ministry of Health and Welfare and the Financial Social Worker Center of Fu-Jen University will need to be continually assessed and improved. Social workers in Taiwan can play a role in increasing financial literacy through a financial capability approach (Collins & Birkenmaier, 2013).

Conclusion

Using CFEDAs as an example, this article analyses child poverty in Taiwan and the process of passing a policy to alleviate it. It discusses how political agenda setting cannot be initiated all at once. Rather, it involves a long-term converging process of three policy streams: problem, policy and politics. When these three streams converged in Taiwan, a policy window opened, allowing CFEDAs onto the political agenda and paving the way for a an eventual policy action.

On 6 June 2018, President Tsai, Ing-wen completed the culmination of that policy action by signing into law the first anti-poverty policy in Taiwan developed to provide incentives for the poor to save for their future, gain access to financial information and make investments in a planned way. The policy will involve an allocated public spending up to 26.1 billion within 18-year period. In the future, it will take an administration's strong will and commitment to allocate the necessary resources to the policy. In a press announcement, President Tsai, Ing-wen said she, 'would ensure the program receives sufficient funding', adding that, 'it is the government's responsibility to guarantee equal opportunity for all'.

Disclosure statement

No potential conflict of interest was reported by the author.

References

Adams, D., & Beverly, S. (2013). Low-income parents of preschool children: Financial knowledge, attitudes, behaviors, and ownership. In J. Birkenmaier, M. Sherraden, & J. Curley (Eds.), *Financial capability and asset development: Research, education, policy, and practice* (pp. 108–128). New York, NY: Oxford University Press.

Beverly, S. G., & Sherraden, M. (1999). Institutional determinants of saving: Implications for low-income households and public policy. *Journal of Socio-Economics*, 28(4), 457–473.

Bradbury, B. (2003). Child poverty: A review. *FaHCSIA Social Policy Research Paper No. 20*. doi:10.2139/ssrn.1729524.

Chang, Y. C. (1993). *Assets accumulation among low-income families*. (Dissertation). Mandel School of Applied Social Science, Case Western Reserve University.

Cheng, L. (2003). *Developing family development accounts in Taipei: Policy innovation from income to assets (CSD Working Paper 03–09)*. St. Louis, MO: Washington University, Center for Social Development.

Cheng, L. C. (2000). *The report on feasibility evaluation of Taipei Development Accounts for low-income families*. Taipei: Taipei City Government Printing Office.

Collins, J. M., & Birkenmaier, J. (2013). Building the capacity of social workers to enhance financial capability. In J. Birkenmaier, M. Sherraden, & J. Curley (Eds.), *Financial capability and asset development: Research, education, policy, and practice* (pp. 302–322). New York, NY: Oxford University Press.

Dahlman, C. J., & Sanaikone, O. (1997). Taiwan, China: Policies and institutions for rapid growth. In D. M. Leipziger (Ed.), *Lessens from East Asia* (pp. 83–154). Ann Arbor, MI: The University of Michigan Press.

Duncan, G. J., & Brooks-Gunn, J. (1997). *Consequences of growing up poor*. New York, NY: Russell Sage Foundation.

Haggard, S. (2001). Institutions and globalization: The aftermath of the Asian financial crisis. *American Asian Review*, 19(2), 71–98.

Kingdon, J. W. (1986). *Agendas, alternatives, and public policies* (2nd ed.). New York, NY: Longman.

Krongkaew, M. (2002). Social consequences of the East Asian economic crisis: A case of globalization gone wrong. In K. T. Lee (Ed.), *Globalization and the Asia Pacific Economy* (pp. 60–84). London, UK: Routledge.

Kuo, D. J., Wang, Y. C., Chen, C. C., Hsiu, T. H., Chen, S. J., Tzen, Y. J., & Chang, Y. J. (2013). Effects of economic burden on long-term aspirations of health administration graduates. *Journal of Tzu Chi University of Science and Technology*, 20, 21–44.

Lee, K. T. (2002). Introduction. In K. T. Lee (Ed.), *Globalization and the Asia Pacific Economy* (pp. 1–6). London, UK: Routledge.

Lee, S., & Wang, T. (2011). Developing temporal changes in Taiwanese child poverty rate with Das Gupta's method. *Tamkang Journal of Humanities and Social Science*, 48, 125–159.

Leu, C., Chen, K., & Chen, H. (2016). A multidimensional approach to child poverty in Taiwan. *Children and Youth Services Review*, 66, 35–44.

McDaniel, B. A. (2000). A survey on entrepreneurship and innovation. *The Social Science Journal, 37*(2), 277–284.

Ministry of Education. (2018). The statistics of student loan, provided by the department of higher education. Retrieved from http://stats.moe.gov.tw/files/important/OVERVIEW_F03.pdf

Ministry of Health and Welfare. (2018, August 5). Child and Youth Welfare Institutions and Services. Retrieved from https://dep.mohw.gov.tw/DOS/lp-2974-113.html

Mintrom, M. (2000). *Policy entrepreneurs and school choice.* Washington, DC: Georgetown University Press.

National Development Council. (2014). *Population projections 2014–2050.* Taipei, Taiwan: Government Printing Office of Republic of China. ISBN13: 9789860419573

Sherraden, M. (1991). *Assets and the poor: A new American welfare policy.* Armonk, NY: M. E. Sharpe.

Sherraden, M. (2001). Asset-building policy and programs for the poor. In T. M. Shapiro & E. N. Wolff (Eds.), Chapter 9: *Assets for the poor: The benefits of spreading asset ownership* (pp. 302–323). New York, NY: Russell Sage Foundation.

Sun, C. C. (1995). *Analyzing the development of social assistance in Taiwan.* Taipei, Taiwan: Shih-Ying Publisher.

Yang, T. (2015). Why economic development in Taiwan grew, but salary went down? Retrieved from http://research.sinica.edu.tw/taiwan-economic-salary-yang-tzu-ting

Zou, L., Cheng, L., Lee, E., Teyra, C., Chen, C., & Song, S. S. (2013). A comparative study on asset-building policy diffusion in Korea and Taiwan. *China Journal of Social Work, 6*(2), 149–162.

Assessing the impact of an asset-based intervention on educational outcomes of orphaned children and adolescents: findings from a randomised experiment in Uganda

Proscovia Nabunya, Phionah Namatovu, Christopher Damulira, Apollo Kivumbi, William Byansi, Miriam Mukasa, Jennifer Nattabi and Fred M. Ssewamala

ABSTRACT

This paper examines the effect of an asset-based intervention on academic performance and school transition among orphaned and vulnerable children in Uganda. Participants were randomly assigned to either the control arm or two treatment arms receiving an asset-based intervention. Participants in the treatment arms scored better grades; and had higher odds of transitioning to post-primary education relative to the control arm. Programmes which target financial insecurity may have a positive impact on the educational achievement and progression of orphaned children. There is a need to consider incorporating asset-based interventions within the development of educational policy, especially in low-income countries.

Introduction

Approximately 50 million children in sub-Saharan Africa (SSA) are orphans, i.e. have lost one or both biological parents; more than 15 million of these have lost their parent(s) to HIV/AIDS (UNICEF, 2016). In Uganda, one of the SSA countries hardest hit by the epidemic, more than 1.2 million children are orphaned as a direct result of the disease (UNICEF, 2016). Children orphaned as a result of HIV/AIDS are at a greater risk of poor schooling and educational outcomes compared to non-orphans and children orphaned due to other causes (Bicego, Rutstein, & Johnson, 2003; Case, Paxton, & Ableidinger, 2004). They are more likely to have poor educational outcomes, including lower school enrolment and attendance rates, less likely to be at a proper education level and are more likely to drop out of school completely (Case et al., 2004; Evan & Miguel, 2004; Kasirye & Hisali, 2010; Monasch & Boerma, 2004).

Given the aforementioned risks, educational opportunities are a key component of the current safety net programmes for orphaned and vulnerable children (OVCs) in communities heavily affected by HIV/AIDS (Hunter & Williamson, 2000). Indeed, OVCs are widely considered a subset of the population targeted by Education for All – a Dakar Framework for Action global commitment that obligates countries to ensure that all children (especially girls, children in difficult circumstances and ethnic minorities) have access to and complete, free and compulsory primary education of good quality (UNESCO, 2000).

Uganda is one of the countries that embraced the Education for All movement. In 1997, Universal Primary Education (UPE), was instituted as one of the United Nations Millennium Development Goals, wherein each child of school-going age is allowed to attend primary school without paying tuition. The abolition of school fees improved entry into primary schooling, incentivised school enrolment and reduced dropout, particularly for girls and for children in rural areas (Deininger, 2003; Grogan, 2009). Between 2000 and 2015, access to primary school increased by 27.7%, and net enrollment at primary school level increased from 83% to 96% (MoES, 2015). However, the completion rates (i.e. the percentage of students of official graduation age who complete primary school) remains lower than the 100% target (Uganda Ministry of Education and Sports [MoES], 2015). The 2016/2017 statistics from MoES indicate that the survival rate to primary seven (i.e. the percentage of a cohort of students enrolled in a given year who reach primary seven) was only 32%, and out of these only 62% were able to complete primary education (i.e. sit for their Primary Leaving Examinations [PLE]) (MoES, 2017).

Despite progress in school access and enrolment, Uganda still faces challenges in ensuring that OVCs participate in and complete primary schooling. The challenges include lack of infrastructure (e.g. classrooms and sanitation facilities given high enrolment rates), high dropout rates (especially among girls), teacher absenteeism and high attrition rates, and the HIV/AIDS epidemic that affect both the supply of qualified teachers and school participation of OVCs (MoES, 2015). These challenges, combined with poor schooling and educational outcomes associated with HIV orphanhood (Bicego, et al., 2003; Case et al., 2004), further limit the opportunities of OVCs from benefiting from the education policy of education for all.

Improving household economic security and providing psychosocial support to affected children and their caregivers is one strategy to address the needs of OVCs. There has been a growing interest in asset-building interventions to enable individuals with limited financial and economic resources or opportunities to acquire and accumulate long-term productive assets (Ssewamala, 2015). Asset-based interventions are modelled on *asset theory* (Sherraden, 1990, 1991), which posits that assets (e.g. savings, educational opportunities, economic opportunities, including microenterprise activities) have important social, economic and psychological benefits for individuals and families. In addition, Sherraden theorises that holding even minor financial or material assets affects individuals' behaviours, attitudes and hopes for the future. The acquisition of assets creates a sense of financial security, which in turn improves self-confidence, responsibility and hope for the future. This is what Schreiner and Sherraden (2007) refer to as *asset effects*.

Several studies both in the developed and developing world have demonstrated positive outcomes, ranging from improved health and psychosocial outcomes, financial outcomes and social outcomes, including educational outcomes (Adato & Bassett, 2009; Cheatham & Elliott, 2013; Curley, Ssewamala, & Han, 2010; Elliott, 2009; Han, Ssewamala, & Wang, 2013; Kim & Sherraden, 2011; Ssewamala, Han, Neilands, Ismayilova, & Sperber, 2010; Ssewamala & Ismayilova, 2009; Ssewamala, Neilands, Waldfogel, & Ismayilova, 2012). For example, previous studies among OVCs in Uganda found that participating in asset-based interventions, specifically those that use matched savings accounts, was associated with positive changes in adolescents' future educational planning, higher levels of confidence in the future, better school grades and school attendance (Curley et al., 2010; Ssewamala & Ismayilova, 2009). Therefore, asset-based interventions have the potential to increase household economic resources and reduce economic stressors associated with paying non-tuition requirements, thereby reducing student's absenteeism and improving their performance in school.

Although the aforementioned studies documented positive school outcomes and educational planning among OVCs in Uganda, they have all been tested using relatively small samples, with relatively short intervention and follow-up periods. In addition, none examined participants' transition rates and progression from primary school to post-primary education. Yet, post-primary education is equally important in defining children's career paths and preparing them for futures that contribute to a country's economic, political and social development. This paper, therefore, examines the impact of an asset-based intervention on academic performance and school transition among a relatively large sample of OVCs, using longitudinal data collected over 5 years, and comparing three study groups. In implementing UPE, this specific focus is important to researchers developing strategies to address the challenges associated with educational outcomes of OVCs in SSA countries heavily affected by HIV/AIDS.

Methods

Study sample and design

This paper uses data from the *Bridges to the Future* study (hereafter *Bridges* study), a 5-year (2011–2016) randomised controlled trial funded by the National Institute of Child Health and Human Development (NICHD Grant #1R01 HD070727-01, PI: Fred Ssewamala, PhD).

The *Bridges* study evaluated the impact of a family asset-based intervention that use Child Development Accounts (CDAs) on the developmental outcomes of OVCs in Southern Uganda. Forty-eight primary schools were randomly assigned to either the control arm (n = 16 schools, 496 participants) or one of the two treatment arms: *Bridges* arm (n = 16 schools, 402 participants) or *Bridges Plus* arm (n = 16 schools, 512 participants). Eligible participants had lost one or both biological parents to HIV/AIDS, lived within a family and not an institution, and were in grades 5 or 6 of a public primary school. Participants in the control condition received 'usual care' services offered to OVCs in the region, including food aid and scholastic materials. Participants in the two treatment arms (*Bridges* and *Bridges Plus*) received usual care services plus the following intervention components: A matched savings account in a form of a CDA with a matching rate of 1:1 for the *Bridges* arm or a 2:1 match ratio for the *Bridges Plus* arm; microenterprise workshops for participants and their caregivers; and a one-hour monthly mentorship programme for participants. Additional information on the Suubi and Bridges mentorship programme has been published elsewhere (Nabunya, Ssewamala, Mukasa, Byansi, & Nattabi, 2015; Ssewamala, Nabunya, Mukasa, Ilic, & Nattabi, 2014).

Measures

Data for the Bridges study were collected at baseline, 12, 24, 36, and 48 months post baseline. Each study participant responded to a 90-min survey administered by trained Ugandan interviewers. The primary outcomes for this analysis were OVCs' academic performance and school transition, collected between 24- and 48-months follow-ups.

Academic performance was measured using official scores from PLE, a national standardised examination administered by the MoES to all students completing primary school in Uganda. All students intending to enroll in post-primary education including vocational institutions must complete and pass the PLE. Participants in the *Bridges* study were recruited within their last 3 years of primary schooling; therefore, their PLE scores were collected between 24 and 48 months follow-ups. PLE scores are measured in aggregates, ranging from 4 (best) to 36 (worst). To illustrate, a total aggregate of 4 means that a child received Distinction 1 (also presented at D1, the best grade one could get in any given subject) for each of the four subjects on which each student is tested (i.e. English Mathematics, Social Studies, Science). Likewise, if a child gets a total aggregate of 36, it means that he/she got Failure 9 (also presented as F9, the worst grade one could get) for each of the four subjects outlined above.

School transition was measured by participants' enrollment into post-primary education, (i.e. secondary/high school or vocational institutions). This data was collected between 24- and 48-months follow-up. Responses were coded as '1' for those who had transitioned to post-primary education and '0' for those who had not transitioned.

The independent variable was participation in the *Bridges* intervention. Participants' demographic and household characteristics included as control variables were age, gender, orphanhood status (single or double orphan), the child's primary caregiver, household size, family cohesion, availability of personal savings and household assets. A household asset index was created, measuring the amount of assets (ranging from 0 to 20 items) reported by participants in the form of home ownership, land or rental property, means of transportation, gardens and livestock, and any ownership of a family microenterprise business.

Data analysis

Baseline sample characteristics were analysed and compared between the three study arms (i.e. the control arm, *Bridges* arm, *Bridges Plus* arm). Specifically, chi-square tests of independence and analysis of variance (ANOVA) were conducted. A descriptive analysis of school outcomes (i.e. PLE performance and school transition to post-primary education) was conducted. In addition, ordinary least squares regression analysis was conducted to examine the effect of the intervention on academic performance (PLE scores). Binary logistic regression analysis was conducted to examine the effect of the intervention on school transition. In both regression models, we controlled for participants' demographics and household characteristics.

Results

Characteristics of the study sample

Baseline sample characteristics are summarised in Table 1. The average age of participants was 12.7 years. The majority of participants were female (56%). Across all three study arms, participants reported statistically different distribution on orphanhood status, with a higher likelihood of being paternal orphans (i.e. had lost a biological father) ($\chi^2 = 10.27$, $p \leq .05$). Participants lived in households with an average of six members, with three children under the age of 18 years. About 39% of participants reported a surviving biological parent as their primary caregiver and 37% reported their grandparents. The average score of family cohesion was 23.5 (SD = 5.13), indicating a moderate level of family closeness. In terms of household assets, the average asset ownership reported was 9.73 items out of the possible 20, indicating moderate levels of household asset ownership. The majority of participants (69%) reported no personal savings.

PLE performance and school transition

Descriptive analysis results of school outcomes are provided in Table 2. Of the total sample, about 61% completed their PLE, meaning that they completed their primary education. Participants in both treatment arms completed PLE at similar rates, higher than those in the control arm. The average PLE aggregate score was 24.57, with participants in the *Bridges* arm (mean score = 22.6) performing better compared to their counterparts in the *Bridges Plus* arm (mean score = 24.33) and the control arm (mean score = 26.74). In terms of school transition, about 46% of the total sample (representing

Table 1. Baseline sample characteristics: n (%).

Variable	Total sample (N = 1410)	Bridges Plus arm (n = 512)	Bridges arm (n = 402)	Control arm (n = 496)	F-value or χ^2
Participants' characteristics					
Age (mean, SD)	12.70 (1.26)	12.71 (1.24)	12.56 (1.31)	12.75 (1.23)	2.74
Gender					0.28
Female	789 (55.96)	288 (56.25)	228 (56.72)	273 (55.04)	
Male	621 (44.04)	224 (43.75)	174 (43.28)	223 (44.96)	
Orphan-hood status					10.57*
Double orphan	297 (21.06)	104 (20.31)	70 (17.41)	123 (24.80)	
Maternal orphan	302 (21.42)	113 (22.07)	79 (19.65)	110 (22.18)	
Paternal orphan	811 (57.52)	295 (57.62)	253 (62.94)	263 (53.02)	
Household characteristics					
Number of people in the household (mean, SD)	6.35 (2.79)	6.32 (2.73)	6.26 (2.62)	6.47 (2.97)	0.67
Number of children in the household (mean, SD)	3.18 (2.20)	3.22 (2.17)	3.11 (2.09)	3.20 (2.32)	0.34
Family assets (mean, SD)	9.73 (3.22)	9.79 (3.29)	9.52 (3.26)	9.83 (3.12)	1.16
Family cohesion (mean, SD)	23.50 (5.13)	23.39 (5.06)	23.27 (5.02)	23.80 (5.27)	1.40
Availability of personal savings					3.35
Yes	433 (30.71)	172 (33.59)	120 (29.85)	141 (28.43)	
No	977 (69.26)	340 (66.41)	282 (70.15)	355 (71.57)	
Caregiver type					6.59
Biological parent	552 (39.15)	216 (42.19)	160 (39.80)	176 (35.48)	
Grandparent(s)	516 (36.60)	182 (35.55)	137 (34.08)	197 (39.72)	
Other relatives (i.e. *aunt, uncle, siblings, in-laws*)	342 (24.26)	114 (22.27)	105 (26.12)	123 (24.80)	

Table 2. Descriptive analysis of PLE performance and school transition: n (%).

Variables	Total (N = 1410)	Bridges Plus arm (n = 512)	Bridges arm (n = 402)	Control arm (n = 496)
Completed PLE				
Yes	856 (60.71)	319 (62.30)	264 (65.67)	273 (55.04)
No	554 (39.29)	193 (37.70)	138 (34.33)	223 (44.96)
PLE scores (mean, SD)	24.57 (6.98)	24.33 (6.24)	22.62 (7.78)	26.74 (6.39)
Transitioned to post-primary				
% of the sample	571 (45.86)	224 (50.56)	187 (51.80)	160 (36.28)
% of those who completed PLE	571 (66.7)	224 (70.2)	187 (70.8)	160 (71.7)
Dropped out of school	633 (44.9)	204 (39.8)	162 (40.3)	267 (53.8)
Repeated a grade/still in primary school	41 (2.9)	15 (2.9)	12 (3.0)	14 (2.8)
Lost to follow-up	165 (11.7)	18 (3.5)	12 (3.0)	55 (11.1)

about 67% of those who completed PLE) transitioned to post-primary school. About half of participants in both *Bridges* and *Bridges Plus* arms transitioned to post-primary education, compared to only 36% of participants in the control arm. Overall, participants who completed PLE had a high likelihood of transitioning to post-primary education.

Finally, at 48-months follow-up, 59% (n = 839) of participants had not transitioned to post-primary education. They had either dropped out of school before or after completing primary school (44.9%), had not completed primary school at the time of interviews (2.9%), or lost to follow up (11.7%). Results from regression analyses are presented in the next section.

Effect of the bridges intervention on academic performance and school transition

Table 3 illustrates the effect of the *Bridges* intervention on participants' PLE scores and school transition. Results indicate that participating in an asset-based intervention (*Bridges* or *Bridges Plus*) was associated with better PLE grades (lower scores indicate better performance) and transitioning to post-primary education. Specifically, controlling for participants' demographic and household characteristics (model 1), participants in the *Bridges* arm ($b = -3.78$, 95% confidence interval [CI] = $-4.92, -2.64$, $p \leq 0.001$) and *Bridges Plus* arm ($b = -2.23$, 95% CI = $-3.32, -1.13$, $p \leq 0.001$), were more likely to report better PLE scores compared to participants in the control condition. Between the intervention groups, participants in the *Bridges* arm, receiving the 1:1 match rate, scored 1.55-point higher than those in the *Bridges Plus* arm receiving 1:2 match rate. Participants' gender ($b = 1.25$, 95% CI = 0.29, 2.22, $p \leq 0.01$), participants' age ($b = 0.98$, 95% CI = 0.59, 1.36, $p \leq 0.001$) and family assets ($b = 0.28$, 95% CI = 0.14, 0.43, $p \leq 0.001$) were inversely associated with PLE grades.

Similarly, participants receiving the intervention exhibited higher odds of transitioning to post-primary education (model 2). Specifically, the odds of transitioning to post-primary education were 1.69 times higher for *Bridges* arm participants (odds ratio [OR] = 1.69, 95% CI = 1.27, 2.25, $p \leq 0.001$) and 1.66 times higher for *Bridges Plus* arm participants (OR = 1.66, 95% CI = 1.28, 2.18, $p \leq 0.001$), relative to the control condition. In addition, participants who identified as paternal orphans (OR = 1.42, 95% CI = 1.02, 1.98, $p \leq 0.05$), and those reporting more individuals living in the household (OR = 1.09, 95% CI = 1.01, 1.19, $p \leq 0.05$) had higher odds of transitioning to post-primary education. However, older adolescents had lower odds of transitioning to post-primary education compared to younger adolescents (OR = 0.64, 95% CI = 0.58, 0.71, $p \leq 0.001$).

Table 3. Regression models on PLE scores and school transition.

Variables	Model 1: PLE scores: b (95% CI)	Model 2: School transition: OR (95% CI)
Intervention (control)		
Bridges	−3.78 (−4.92, −2.64)***	1.69 (1.27, 2.25)***
Bridges Plus	−2.23 (−3.32, −1.13)***	1.66 (1.28, 2.18)***
Participants' characteristics		
Age	0.98 (0.59, 1.36)***	0.64 (0.58, 0.71)***
Gender (female)	1.25 (0.29, 2.22)**	1.04 (0.82, 1.32)
Orphan hood (double orphan)		
Maternal orphan	−0.46 (−1.93, 1.02)	1.41 (0.98, 2.04)
Paternal orphan	0.12 (−1.19, 1.43)	1.42 (1.02, 1.98)*
Household characteristics		
Number of people in the household	0.004 (−0.33, 0.34)	1.09 (1.01, 1.19)*
Number of children in the household	−0.009 (−0.43, 0.42)	0.92 (0.78, 1.29)
Family assets	0.28 (0.14, 0.43)***	1.00 (0.96, 1.04)
Family cohesion	0.03 (−0.06, 0.12)	1.00 (0.98, 1.03)
Availability of personal savings	0.48 (−0.54, 1.49)	1.01 (0.78, 1.29)
Caregiver (others)		
Biological parent	−0.89 (−2.15, 0.38)	1.09 (0.79, 1.52)
Grandparent	−0.23 (−1.43, 0.96)	0.86 (0.63, 1.16)
F or χ^2	7.64***	131.23***
df	13	13
Adjusted R^2	0.09	0.07
N	856	1375

*$p \leq .05$; **$p \leq .01$; ***$p \leq .001$.

Discussion

This paper examines the effects of participating in an asset-based intervention on educational outcomes (i.e. academic performance and school transition from primary to post-primary education) of OVCs in Uganda. Over the 5-year assessment period, the *Bridges* intervention, which combines CDAs, a mentorship programme and financial planning and microenterprise development workshops, indicate positive outcomes for OVCs. Results show that OVCs receiving the intervention (i.e. *Bridges* and *Bridges Plus* arms) performed significantly better on the PLE and had higher odds of transitioning to secondary/high school or vocational institutions than their counterparts in the control arm. Because OVCs receiving the intervention (and their families) did not have to worry about paying the entirety of an expensive post-primary education, it could be that they were more likely to think beyond primary school education and concentrate on their studies to qualify and enrol in post-primary education. Moreover, given that participants receiving the intervention met with peer mentors throughout the intervention period to discuss academic planning, setting realistic academic and career goals, financial planning and asset accumulation, it is possible that adolescents were able to integrate the knowledge and skills acquired during their mentorship sessions into their schooling, leading to better performance.

The findings of this study support the premise of asset theory that guides the design and implementation of this work. In particular, promoting and increasing the economic assets and opportunities of vulnerable youth, such as OVCs, encourages more positive beliefs and attitudes about the future (Schreiner & Sherraden, 2007; Sherraden, 1991, 1990). In this case, the multicomponent intervention provided a sense of economic security through the provision of matched savings, provided OVCs with a sense of hope to complete primary school without economic constraints, enabling them to envision a more tangible and realistic future, as well as personal responsibility of paying attention in class and working harder to achieve better grades. These findings are also consistent with previous findings that documented positive impacts on academic participation in terms of attendance, academic planning and performance in Uganda (Curley, Ssewamala, Nabunya, Ilic, & Keun, 2014; Ssewamala & Curley, 2006; Ssewamala & Ismayilova, 2009).

In addition, though study participants were recruited during their last 2–3 years of primary schooling, a large number of participants had either dropped out of school completely or were still in primary school 5 years later. Among those who had dropped out, more than half (53.8%) were participants in the control condition. This finding is consistent with those reported by Kasirye and Hisali (2010), wherein orphans from poor families affected by HIV/AIDS were more likely to fall 3 years behind their appropriate grade level compared to non-orphans. This situation may be attributed to several factors beyond the intervention, such as family responsibilities, grade repetition/falling behind, and change of residences, which are common among OVCs, as well as stigma and discrimination associated with HIV/AIDS and orphanhood. Specifically, issues of family responsibilities that force OVCs to take on additional household responsibilities in lieu of schooling remains a major challenge to educational participation and achievement in Uganda, and many parts of SSA (Nabunya & Ssewamala, 2014). Low levels of school attendance and participation inhibit children's performance in school and ultimately lead to grade repetition and school dropout. In addition, OVCs are more likely to bounce from one extended family to another, especially when the current family is overwhelmed with a large number of orphaned children and poverty. In such cases, children are often forced to change schools, which results in setbacks in schooling and performance.

Furthermore, though participants were enrolled in UPE with no school fees required, schools continue to experience inadequate supplies and infrastructures, including instructional materials, classrooms, gender-specific bathrooms and teachers. Schools often shift the burden of paying for these infrastructures to parents and caregivers in the form of 'building fees.' This often becomes the basis for sending children back home for lack of payments, leading to missed schooling, poor performance and eventually dropping out. All these situations combined might help explain why a number of participants in our study had not transitioned from primary school.

Study limitations

Given that the intervention was provided as a bundle of services that included matched savings, mentorship, financial planning and microenterprise development, it is not possible to measure the unique contribution of each individual component on educational outcomes. Future research should consider testing the effectiveness of each of the intervention components on OVC outcomes. Also, the lack of a true control condition may have implications for findings. Researchers should consider designs, wherein non-intervention participants do not receive support services from the study to ascertain the net effect of the intervention. The sample was limited to rural school/participants. Findings could be different among schools and participants in an urban school setting.

Implications and conclusion

Even with these limitations, the findings indicate that participating in an economic intervention has the potential to improve OVCs' academic performance and reduce their economic barriers to transition from primary education to secondary school or vocational education. The small differences observed between the two intervention groups have implications for programming and policy. Specifically, programmes intending to incorporate matched saving interventions within the social protection efforts for OVCs may not need to select a higher match rate to see positive results. Even small financial contributions can offset the possible negative outcomes for OVCs, especially those orphaned as a result of HIV/AIDS. Finally, outcomes of national policies such as UPE could be improved and strengthened by incorporating economic strengthening components to help address poverty issues for poor families, especially those caring for OVCs to offset their human capital outcomes, including educational achievement.

Disclosure statement

No potential conflict of interest was reported by the authors.

Funding

This work was supported by the Eunice Kennedy Shriver National Institute of Child Health and Human Development [1R01 HD070727-01].

References

Adato, M., & Bassett, L. (2009). Social protection to support vulnerable children and families: The potential of cash transfers to protect education, health and nutrition. *AIDS Care, 21*(S1), 60–75.

Bicego, G., Rutstein, S., & Johnson, K. (2003). Dimensions of the emerging orphan crisis in sub-Saharan Africa. *Social Science & Medicine, 56*(6), 1235–1247.

Case, A., Paxton, C., & Ableidinger, J. (2004). Orphans in Africa: Parental death, poverty, and school enrollment. *Demography, 41*, 483–508.

Cheatham, G. A., & Elliott, W. (2013). The effects of family college savings on postsecondary school enrollment rates of students with disabilities. *Economics of Education Review, 33*, 95–111.

Curley, J., Ssewamala, F., & Han, C. (2010). Assets and educational outcomes: Child Development Accounts (CDAs) for orphaned children in Uganda. *Children and Youth Services Review, 32*(11), 1585–1590.

Curley, J., Ssewamala, F. M., Nabunya, P., Ilic, V., & Keun, H. C. (2014). Child Development Accounts (CDAs): An asset building strategy to empower girls in Uganda. *International Social Work*. doi:10.1177/0020872813508569

Deininger, K. (2003). Does cost of schooling affect enrollment by the poor? Universal primary education in Uganda. *Economics of Education Review, 22*(3), 291–305.

Elliott, W. (2009). Children's college aspirations and expectations: The potential role of children's development accounts (CDAs). *Children and Youth Services Review, 31*, 274–283.

Evan, D., & Miguel, E. (2004). Orphans and schooling in Africa: A longitudinal analysis. *Demography, 44*(1), 33–57.

Grogan, L. (2009). Universal primary education and school entry in Uganda. *Journal of African Economies, 18*(2), 183–211.

Han, C.-K., Ssewamala, F. M., & Wang, J. S.-H. (2013). Family economic empowerment and mental health among AIDS-affected children living in AIDS-impacted communities: Evidence from a randomized evaluation in Southwestern Uganda. *Journal of Epidemiology and Community Health, 67*(3), 225–230.

Hunter, S., & Williamson, J. (2000). *Children on the brink: Strategies to support a generation isolated by HIV/AIDS*. Washington, DC: USAID.

Kasirye, I., & Hisali, E. (2010). The socioeconomic impact of HIV/AIDS on education outcomes in Uganda: School enrolment and the schooling gap in 2002/2003. *International Journal of Educational Development, 30*, 12–22.

Kim, Y., & Sherraden, M. (2011). Do parental assets matter for children's educational? Attainment? Evidence from mediation tests. *Children and Youth Services Review, 33*, 969–979.

Monasch, R., & Boerma, J. T. (2004). Orphanhood and childcare patterns in sub-Saharan Africa: An analysis of national surveys from 40 countries. *AIDS, 18*, S55–S65.

Nabunya, P., & Ssewamala, F. M. (2014). The effects of parental loss on the psychosocial wellbeing of AIDS-orphaned children living in AIDS-impacted communities: Does gender matter? *Children and Youth Services Review, 43*, 131–137.

Nabunya, P., Ssewamala, F. M., Mukasa, M. N., Byansi, W., & Nattabi, J. (2015). Peer mentorship program on HIV/AIDS knowledge, beliefs, and prevention attitudes among orphaned adolescents: An evidence based practice. *Vulnerable Children and Youth Studies, 10*(4), 345–356.

Schreiner, M., & Sherraden, M. (2007). *Can the poor save? Saving & asset building in individual development accounts*. Piscataway, NJ: Transaction Publishers.

Sherraden, M. (1990). Stakeholding: Notes in a theory of welfare based on assets. *Social Service Review, 64*(4), 580–601.

Sherraden, M. (1991). *Assets and the poor: A new American welfare policy*. New York, NY: M. E. Sharpe.

Ssewamala, F., Nabunya, P., Mukasa, N. M., Ilic, V., & Nattabi, J. (2014). Integrating a mentorship component in programming for care and support of AIDS-orphaned and vulnerable children: Lessons from the suubi and bridges programs in sub-Saharan Africa. *Global Social Welfare, 1*(1), 9–24.

Ssewamala, F. M. (2015). Optimizing the "demographic dividend" in young developing countries: The role of contractual savings and insurance for financing education. *International Journal of Social Welfare, 24*(3), 248–262.

Ssewamala, F. M., & Curley, J. (2006). Asset ownership and school attendance of orphaned children in sub-Saharan Africa. *Social Development Issues, 28*(2), 84–105.

Ssewamala, F. M., Han, C.-K., Neilands, T. B., Ismayilova, L., & Sperber, E. (2010). Effect of economic assets on sexual risk taking intentions among orphaned adolescents in Uganda. *American Journal of Public Health, 100*(3), 483–488.

Ssewamala, F. M., & Ismayilova, L. (2009). Integrating children savings accounts in the care and support of orphaned adolescents in rural Uganda. *Social Service Review, 83*(3), 453–472.

Ssewamala, F. M., Neilands, T. B., Waldfogel, J., & Ismayilova, L. (2012). The impact of a comprehensive microfinance intervention on depression levels of AIDS-orphaned children in Uganda. *Journal of Adolescent Health, 50*(4), 346–352.

Uganda Ministry of Education and Sports [MoES]. (2015). Education for all 2015 national review. Retrieved from http://unesdoc.unesco.org/images/0023/002317/231727e.pdf

Uganda Ministry of Education and Sports [MoES]. (2017). The education and sports sector annual performance report. Financial Year 2016/17. Retrieved from http://www.education.go.ug/files/downloads/ESSAPR%20%202016-17.pdf

UNESCO. (2000). The Dakar Framework for Action. Education for All: Meeting our collective commitment. Retrieved from http://unesdoc.unesco.org/images/0012/001211/121147e.pdf

UNICEF. (2016). The State of the World's Children 2016: A fair chance for every child. Retrieved from http://www.unicef.org/publications/files/UNICEF_SOWC_2016.pdf

A qualitative study on participants' perceptions of child development accounts in Korea

Chang-Keun Han

ABSTRACT

In 2007, Korea implemented Child Development Accounts (CDAs) for institutionalised children in child welfare systems. Since then, the target group and a matching cap of CDAs in Korea have evolved. The target group expanded to include poor children receiving welfare, whereas the matching cap increased from KRW 30,000 (US$26.53) to KRW 40,000 (US$35.38), which is matched at a 1:1 rate. Despite the expansion, there is little empirical evidence examining the extent to which CDAs have influenced the life of participants. Using a content analysis method with a sample ($N = 22$), this study examines how CDAs have changed children's mindsets, saving habits, education, future planning and sponsorship. The findings suggest that CDAs have multiple positive influences on children. This study concludes with policy implications for the inclusive and progressive development of CDAs in Korea.

Introduction

In 2016, approximately 6.7% of the children in South Korea (here after Korea) were estimated to live in poverty (i.e. 50% or lower than a median household income; Yeo, 2018). Child welfare systems – group homes, foster care homes and institutional facilities – care for the most disadvantaged children. As of 31 December 2014, 31,558 were under the care of child welfare systems (Nho, Park, & McCarthy, 2017).

Children in child welfare systems and low-income children in Korea may face economic insecurity, emotional maladaptation and uncertainty of future (Yeo, 2018). Under Korean law, children in child welfare systems should leave by the time they reach the age of 18 (Nho et al., 2017). To help them prepare for self-reliance during and after this transition, the Korean Ministry of Health and Welfare introduced an asset-based policy of Child Development Accounts (CDAs; called as *Didimsiat Tongjang* in Korean) in 2007 (Nam & Han, 2010).

As a social investment strategy that emphasises human capital investments, *Didimsiat Tongjang* pioneered matched saving accounts in Korea. Savings accumulated in the CDAs are matched by the Korean government at a 1:1 rate. Though the CDAs were originally targeted towards institutionalised children living in child welfare systems, they were expanded in 2011 to include children receiving welfare. The connection between sponsorship – donations from the civil sector – and CDAs is a key mechanism that makes CDAs possible in Korea.

There are two types of sponsorship in Korea. First, children living under the care of the child welfare system can receive a general sponsorship from donors. They can opt to make deposits from sponsorship into CDA accounts. Children can use the sponsorship for living costs, education fees or saving in CDA accounts. Second, there is a CDA-designated sponsorship, which is used only for deposits in CDAs. The CDAs Supporting Committee (CDASC) collects the CDA-designated sponsorship and distributes the sponsorship to more disadvantaged children who are likely to have low saving performance in CDA accounts (Nam & Han, 2010).

Despite the importance of CDAs in Korea, few scholarly studies that evaluate their performance have been published since their introduction in 2007. In particular, there are few studies examining how children view CDAs and the extent to which CDAs have changed children. This study aims to fill the gap by providing information about how the CDAs have influenced children's life. This study uses essays published by the CDASC – an organisation managing CDAs in Korea – to examine how CDAs have influenced children participants. Given the importance of the pioneering asset-based policy in Korea, a detailed analysis and evaluation will be helpful to enhance the knowledge of how CDAs can continue to progress.

Literature review: does saving matter for children?

Before examining CDAs in the Korean context, we offer context about asset theory and reviews how asset-based saving policies affect children in other countries in this section. *Assets* or *wealth* are liquid and non-liquid assets (Sherraden, 1991). *Asset theory* emphasises that assets can have multiple positive influences on individuals and families (Sherraden, 1991). In addition to buffering the negative impacts of financial hardships (Han & Rothwell, 2014), holding assets can influence psychological mindsets and behaviours for the future (Sherraden, 1991; Yadama & Sherraden, 1996).

More significantly, assets can have positive impacts on child development (Sherraden, 1991). Engendering positive attitudes toward the future, assets are regarded by some children as resources that help their dreams come true (Han, Ssewamala, & Wang, 2013). Previous studies also have found that assets have multiple influences on children's educational performance (Curley, Ssewamala, & Han, 2010), physical health (Ssewamala, Han, & Neilands, 2009), risk-taking behaviours (Ssewamala, Han, Neilands, Ismayilova, & Sperber, 2010) and mental health including self-esteem and depression (Han et al., 2013; Ssewamala et al., 2009, 2010).

Based on asset theory, Individual Development Accounts (IDAs) for the working poor in the United States began in the 1990s. Key features of IDAs included matched deposits; financial education; direct deposit; voluntary saving; and savings goals for housing, starting a small business and investing in education (Schreiner et al., 2001). With public and private funding, IDAs expanded to include disadvantaged populations. Despite the commonly held view that the poor cannot save, participants in IDAs proved otherwise – and the aforementioned key institutional features had significant impacts (Han & Sherraden, 2009; Schreiner et al., 2001).

Though IDAs target the working poor, CDAs specifically help lift low-income children from poverty. In the United States, recent progress of CDAs is noteworthy. For example, SEED for Oklahoma Kids (SEED OK) is a large-scale experiment that tests inclusive and progressive CDAs. It is inclusive in that every participating child receives an automatically opened an account with an initial 'seed' deposit, and progressive in that low-income participants receive savings matches (Sherraden, 2016). Evaluation studies of SEED OK suggest that assets in CDAs have multiple positive influences on children as well as parents: They can enhance parental future orientation and reduce maternal depressive symptoms (Kim, Huang, Sherraden, & Clancy, 2017; Sherraden, 2016) and have positive influence on the social-emotional development of children (Beverly, Kim, Sherraden, Nam, & Clancy, 2015; Sherraden, 2016).

Other countries have since implemented CDA policies. In Uganda, the asset-building program for children SUUBI (meaning hope) targets AIDS-orphans. Despite the notion that AIDS-orphans have difficulties in saving, the orphans participating in SUUBI were found to save (Ssewamala et al., 2009, 2010). A recent evaluation study (Lee, 2016) on Seoul CDAs reports that, as of 2016, 5,518 children have successfully graduated from the program and 7,589 participants maintained their saving and asset holding. The dropout rate is about 24.2% (4,222 out of 17,457 children). A survey with program graduates (N = 257) from Seoul CDAs found that they have experienced positive impacts on child development (95.8%), parents' relationships with children (93.0%), short-term money management (77.3%) and long-term future planning (75.9%) (Lee, 2016).

Reviews on whether assets matter for children strongly suggest that asset building can have an enormous impact on child development. In addition, it should be emphasised that institutional opportunities of saving matter for helping vulnerable children save.

CDAs in Korea: evolution, performance, and sponsorship

This section explores CDAs in the Korean context. It provides an overview of the policy's evolution, performance and sponsorship.

The evolution of CDAs in Korea

The Korean government introduced CDAs for institutionalised children in April 2007. Since then, CDA policy has been reformed to include expanded saving goals, broader target groups and matching caps (Table 1). First, assets in CDAs were originally limited for education, housing, and starting a small business. Reforms in 2008 expanded those goals to include medical and marriage costs.

Second, when they were initiated in 2007, CDAs were targeted at institutionalised children aged 0 to 18 and proposed to expand to 50% of the children in Korea (Nam & Han, 2010), but that goal was not achieved. As a result, in 2011, CDAs were opened up to children receiving welfare aged 12 who was born in 1999. In 2016, the target age group was again changed to children aged 12 (born in 2005) and 13 (born in 2004) to increase the efficacy of the policy.

Table 1. Reforms of Child Development Accounts in Korea.

	2007	2011	2016	2017
Target	Institutionalised children (aged 0 to 18)	Institutionalised children (aged 0 to 18) & children (aged 12) receiving welfare	Institutionalised children (aged 0 to 18) & children (aged 12 & 13) receiving welfare	Same as left
Matching cap (KRW)	30,000	Same as left	Same as left	40,000
Matching rate	1:1	Same as left	Same as left	Same as left
Maximum monthly savings (KRW)	50,000	500,000 (But matching is only for 30,000)	Same as left	Same as left
Saving goals	Housing Small business Education			
	Medical cost (Since 2008) Marriage cost (Since 2008)	Same as left	Same as left	Same as left

Table 2. Performance of saving in CDAs (as of July 2017).

	Total participants		Account holders		Saving rate (%)	Average monthly savings (KRW)	Savers with KRW30K or more (%)
	n	%	n	%			
Institutionalised children	17,270	19.1	12,002	17.0	97.3	46,801	53.2
Children at foster care	14,853	16.4	8,639	12.3	96.2	42,570	44.1
Youth-headed family	589	0.6	85	0.1	94.1	46,558	10.4
Group home children	3,234	3.6	2,382	3.4	95.5	43,148	54.8
Disability institutions	2,978	3.3	1,129	1.6	98.3	24,219	16.4
Back-to-home children	4,629	5.1	2,615	3.7	95.3	27,354	24.5
Welfare children	47,044	51.9	43,563	61.9	79.9	32,994	63.8
Total	90,597	100.0	70,415	100.0	86.3	36,532	54.3

Source: CDASC internal administration data (2017)

Table 3. Performance of sponsorship in CDAs.

	2007	2014	2015	2016	2017
Amount of sponsorship (KRW billion)	0.69	4.19	4.47	5.14	5.45
Number of sponsors	2,583	12,248	12,989	13,443	14,700

Source: Annual report of Child Development Account Supporting Committee (2017)

Third, the monthly matching cap has been increased to KRW40,000 (US$35.38) from KRW30,000 (US$26.53). Though children can save up to KRW500,000 (US $440.49) monthly (because of the high-interest rate for additional savings, children can save more than the matching cap), government matching is limited to KRW40,000.

Performance of saving in CDAs in Korea

This section reports the performance of asset building in CDAs regarding participation levels, average saving rates, average monthly savings and those saving more than the match of KRW30,000 (Table 2).

As of July 2017, 90,597 children have participated in CDAs (Child Development Accounts Supporting Committee [CDASC], 2017). The largest group is children receiving welfare (51.9%), followed by institutionalised children (19.1%), foster care children (16.4%) and back-to-home children (5.1%). Youth-headed families are the smallest with 0.6%. Back-to-home children who first opened CDA in institutions are allowed to maintain the accounts after returning home. The number of account holders, as of July 2017, is 70,415; the difference between total participants and account holders can be explained by graduates and dropouts. The inflow of welfare children since 2011 explains the highest percentage (61.9%) of all account holders, followed by institutionalised children (17.0%), children at foster care (12.3%) and back-to-home children (3.7%). Youth-headed families are the lowest at 0.1% (CDASC, 2017).

The average saving rate of accountholders measured by at least one deposit per year is about 86.3%. Children in institutions and disability institutions have the highest saving rates of 97.3% and 98.3%, respectively. This can be explained by sponsorship, which targets children with more risks and disadvantages. Children in welfare families have the lowest saving rate of 79.9%. In general, they manage to save in CDAs without sponsorship (CDASC, 2017).

Regarding average monthly savings, children participating in CDAs save an average of KRW36,532 (US$32.18) per month (CDASC, 2017). Despite the notion that low-income children cannot save, it is noteworthy that the average monthly savings are more than the match cap (KRW30,000). In addition, it should be emphasised that the increase in the matching cap to KRW40,000 in 2017 may explain the average monthly savings among at-risk children.

In terms of the percentage of children saving equal to or higher than KRW30,000, a high variation was reported: 54.3%. About 63.8% of the children receiving welfare are reported to save KRW30,000 or more (CDASC, 2017). However, only 10.1% of the child-headed families were reported to achieve the matching cap (KRW30,000). The percentages of savers with KRW30,000 or more among children at disability institutions and back-to-home children are 16.4% and 24.5%, respectively (CDASC, 2017).

Performance of sponsorship

Another feature of CDAs in Korea is the combination of sponsorship (donations from donors) and saving. As discussed above, there are two types of sponsorship. The government transfers general sponsorships to children, who decide how to use it. Some are willing to save a portion of a general sponsorship into the CDAs. The CDASC publicises a CDA-designated sponsorship and collects donations from citizens. The CDA-designated sponsorship is used only for deposits in CDAs. The combination between sponsorship and CDAs is a unique element that makes CDAs possible in Korea. Sponsorship is crucial to help more disadvantaged children keep saving.

With efforts of the CDASC to increase donations from citizens, the annual amount of CDA-designated sponsorship has been increased from KRW0.69 billion (US$0.61 million) in 2007 to KRW5.45 billion (US$4.81 million) in 2017. The number of sponsors shows a 5.7 times increase from 2,583 to 14,700 (Table 3, CDASC, 2017).

Methods

So far, this study has examined the progress and evolution of asset-based policies focusing on CDAs in Korea. Despite the statistical description of saving performance in CDAs, the experience of children participating in CDAs and details of how CDAs have influenced their life remain unclear. To fill the gap, this study uses participant essays from the essay contests CDASC has held annually since 2013. This study analyses 22 essays published by CDASC between the years 2013 and 2016 (CDASC, 2013, 2014, 2015, 2016).

Sample and data

The information for this study is based on passages from the 22 winning essays. Because the winning essays are much more favourable for CDAs, the contents may be biased. However, analysing the essays will be meaningful to understand how children experience participation in CDAs. The sample consists of 10 males and 12 females. Out of 22 samples, 10 children attended middle school, followed by eight high school students and four primary school students. Nineteen out of 22 sample essays come from orphans (Table 4).

Table 4. Sample description.

Year	Gender		Education status			Number of orphans	Number of essays
	Male	Female	Primary school	Middle school	High school		
2013	1	3	1	1	2	4	4
2014	3	5	1	5	2	6	8
2015	4	1	0	3	2	5	5
2016	2	3	2	1	2	4	5
Total	10	12	4	10	8	19	22

Sources: Child Development Accounts Supporting Committee (2013, 2014, 2015, 2016)

Analysis plan

Using transcripts of essays, this study uses content analysis to identify key themes. Content analysis is based on a systematic reading of the texts, which are assigned labels or codes indicating interesting and meaningful pieces of the content (Creswell, 2013). To increase the reliability of the analysis, this study employed two research assistants who separately analysed the transcripts and compared their analysis results.

Results

The content analyses found several key themes. This section summarises the content analysis findings in terms of general views toward CDAs; how participation helped alleviate stress and anxiety; being socialised into saving and impacts of CDAs on children including education, saving habits, future planning and sponsorship.

Views toward CDAs in general

Many participating children expressed thankfulness to CDAs and sponsors:

> CDAs provides me seed money for my future. I should go out of the facility six years later. When I leave this facility, I may face many difficulties and feel anxious. However, I believe CDAs will be my teacher and angel guiding me to go through them.

–Song, 2013

Other children described CDAs as 'power slowly coming to my life', 'investment for my future', 'CDAs is my friend' and 'dream together with CDAs'. These results indicate that CDAs are very meaningful to children participants. Moreover, CDAs influence their thinking and behaviours in positive ways.

Relief from anxieties and stresses

Orphans age out of out-of-home institutions (e.g. orphanage facilities, foster care homes) when they reach age 18. Leaving an institution is very stressful. A settlement fund facilitates the transition but does not offer enough to ensure self-reliance. In this regard, CDAs provide additional resources for children preparing to leave an institution. For example, two participants reported:

Four years later, I should leave my institution. I need to think about what to do, where to live, what to eat, and so on. These are tsunami of stress. But, I was told that I have CDAs against the tsunami. I can do little but meaningful thing for my future. CDAs is like a sunshine relieving my stresses. So, I'm not afraid of my future. Rather, I can think of my bright future.

–Sung, 2015

I feel, I'm taken care by someone else. With supports from three sponsors, I'm not alone. CDAs helped me change my mindsets and have positive attitudes toward others.

–Kim, 2016

Socialisation for saving: learning from seniors

Saving behaviours can be influenced by others. This study found that socialisation is an important mechanism to facilitate saving in CDAs. Orphans in institutions learn how to prepare to leave an institution from their older siblings' experiences in same institution. For example, one participant explained how she came to understand the importance of saving in CDAs from her sister's experience:

I have a very close sister attending a high school. She told me to save a lot in CDAs. I complained, why should I do save, although she did not. But, it didn't take long to realise the importance of saving in CDAs She left my institutions with not enough money.

–Son, 2013

Another participant's brother offered advice regarding saving in CDAs:

Brothers living with me have only 1 year left before leaving my institution. I have 5 years left. I heard many times that brothers worried about future. Brothers also told me to keep saving in CDAs and to prepare for future.

–Cho, 2015

Positive impacts on education

As in many countries, attending and graduating from college is necessary to secure a desirable job. Therefore, achievement in middle and high schools is a crucial indicator of future success. Children participating in CDAs are at risk; therefore, they may appear less likely to focus on studying. However, this study found that many Korean children participants made efforts to learn actively. For example, one participant reported that having a CDA enabled him to focus on his studies, rather than worrying about the future:

Since I recognised that I have CDAs for my future, I can focus on my study. At the second-year exam in my middle school, I reached 4th out of 220 students. In high school, I played as leaders for many areas such as classroom and extracurricular activities.

–Jung, 2014

Another participant reported how the support of CDAs pushed her to work harder:

I don't want to depend on only CDAs for self-reliance. CDAs is like a buttress pushing me to work hard. I should study hard and pass qualifying exams for certificates including computer skills, word process, and audit.

–Lim, 2015

Positive impacts on saving habits

In addition to saving in CDAs, participation taught children enough about saving to inspire them to save voluntarily. In addition to the CDAs, a few children opened regular saving accounts. For example, one student reported applying for scholarships:

This semester, I applied for Samsung Dream Scholarship and received KRW2.4million. Because CDAs is a stepping stone for my future, I'm going to save KRW1.4 in CDAs after using KRW1.0million for education fees.

–Jung, 2015

With CDAs, I can focus on learning in present rather than being worry about future. However, I don't want to depend on only CDAs. I personally opened a regular saving account in a bank.

–Jung, 2014

Positive impacts on future planning

Saving in CDAs represents one step toward making children's hopes and dreams within reach. Many children interviewed for this study have very specific plans for their future professions. Many articulated how they plan to apply CDA savings to make that future a reality:

I want to be a social worker. I ask teachers about how to be a good social worker. I also pray to achieve the goal every day.

–Moon, 2016

Since I know I have CDAs, I think about how to use it. For example, if I got a job with a dormitory, then I will use it for college fees. If my job does not provide a dormitory, then I'll use it for housing. Without CDAs, it's not possible to think about these kinds of things.

–Lim, 2015

Future sponsorship

A very common element in the essays is an expression of thankfulness to the sponsors. Many children mention becoming donors for CDA sponsorship in the future. It indicates that children receiving supports from sponsors want to pay back later:

I'd like to donate and volunteer for disadvantaged populations. I'm going to make progress for self-reliance with thankfulness for sponsors.

–Lee, 2016

If possible, I'd like to sponsor to children who make efforts to achieve self-sufficiency. Probably, my sponsors have same thought. So, I'd like to do my best to be a good person. This will be the best thing I can do.

–Lim, 2015

In the future, I'd like to be a sponsor to CDAs. We say, love can be doubled with sharing. Matching in CDAs is like that. My dream is to buy a dinner to the sponsors with money I earn from my job in the future.

–Son, 2013

Discussion

As the first inclusive asset-based policy in Korea, CDAs target institutionalised children and other disadvantaged populations, facilitate saving among children via sponsorship and promote saving over a long time period (18 years). Influenced by the successful implementation of CDAs, central and local governments have kicked off diverse asset-building programs targeting welfare recipients, low-income households and youth (Hong & Han, 2018).

Key findings from this study suggest that CDAs may have multiple positive impacts on children in terms of mindsets, saving habits, education and future planning. These findings are consistent with previous research (Curley et al., 2010; Han et al., 2013; Yadama & Sherraden, 1996). Because many children in the study are orphans and must leave the institutions that have been their home when they reach adulthood, they face high levels of anxiety and stress about the future. This study shows that assets in CDAs may play a significant role in relieving such stress. In addition, CDAs engender in children a positive view toward donation and sponsorship. It is also noteworthy that children who received support from sponsors want to pay back and to donate in the future.

This study provides several policy issues related to the future directions of CDAs. First, the scope of CDAs in Korea should be further expanded. Though reforms expanded CDAs to low-income household children receiving welfare, there are still many children in need of institutional opportunities to save. In particular, the designated target groups by age (age 12 and 13) may hinder the development of inclusive CDAs. Limited budgets explain why the government has taken this selective approach. However, the government should take more inclusive steps to further expand the target group.

Second, policy review should be continuously operated. Currently, the CDASC does not operate on a regular basis. The CDASC should have regular discussions on the policy directions, development of sponsorships, inclusiveness of CDAs and program evaluation of CDAs. Through the systematic policy review, CDASC can make progress for more inclusive CDAs in Korea.

Third, the Moon Jae In administration plans to implement child allowance (Maximum KRW 100,000: US$88.92) to children aged 0 to 5 in September 2018. The proposed allowances can be saved in CDAs. This would allow children at child welfare systems to save up to KRW 140,000 (KRW 100,000 from child allowance and KRW 40,000 from sponsorship), enhancing the saving performance of CDAs.

Fourth, it remains unclear whether children ageing out of institutions achieve self-reliance at age 18. Matched savings in CDAs help but may not be enough to achieve the goal. Since 2006, the Korean government has implemented independent living support programs for children leaving out-home-care facilities. For example, the government provides them housing, college scholarships, and one-time lump sums when they leave the facilities (Nho et al., 2017). Policymakers should re-examine the systematic links among policies supporting children leaving out-home-care facilities.

Conclusion

This is the first study examining the program perception of CDAs children in Korea. Findings suggest that CDAs may provide hope and enhance preparation for the future to children participating in CDAs. Still, many issues remain unstudied. First, it is unknown how much-institutionalised children receiving sponsorships have saved voluntarily. Second, there is little information on how children leaving institutions have used savings from CDAs. Future studies should be developed to fill the gaps. A longitudinal research study following up with their lives will be necessary to examine the long-term impacts of CDAs on children. Because CDAs play significant roles in supporting vulnerable children in positive ways, more inclusive development of CDAs will be necessary.

Disclosure statement

No potential conflict of interest was reported by the author.

References

Beverly, S. G., Kim, Y., Sherraden, M., Nam, Y., & Clancy, M. (2015). Can child development accounts be inclusive? Early evidence from a statewide experiment. *Children and Youth Services Review*, *53*(6), 92–104.

Child Development Accounts Supporting Committee. (2013). *Results of essay competition of child development accounts*. Seoul: CDASC.

Child Development Accounts Supporting Committee. (2014). *Results of essay competition of child development accounts*. Seoul: CDASC.

Child Development Accounts Supporting Committee. (2015). *Results of essay competition of child development accounts*. Seoul: CDASC.

Child Development Accounts Supporting Committee. (2016). *Results of essay competition of child development accounts*. Seoul: CDASC.

Child Development Accounts Supporting Committee. (2017). *Annual report of Child Development Accounts*. Seoul: CDASC.

Creswell, J. W. (2013). *Qualitative inquiry and research design: Choosing among five approaches*. Washington, DC: Sage.

Curley, J., Ssewamala, F., & Han, C.-K. (2010). Assets and educational outcomes: Child Development Accounts (CDAs) for orphaned children in Uganda. *Children and Youth Services Review, 32*(11), 1585–1590.

Han, C.-K., & Rothwell, D. W. (2014). Savings and family functioning during the 2008 recession: An exploratory study with lower income Singaporeans. *International Social Work, 57*(6), 630–644.

Han, C.-K., & Sherraden, M. (2009). Do institutions really matter for saving among low-income households? A comparative approach. *Journal of Socio-Economics, 38*(3), 475–483.

Han, C.-K., Ssewamala, F., & Wang, J. S.-H. (2013). Family economic empowerment and mental health among AIDS-affected children living in AIDS-impacted communities: Evidence from a randomized evaluation in southwestern Uganda. *Journal of Epidemiology & Community Health, 67*(3), 225–230.

Hong, S.-I., & Han, C.-K. (2018). An exploratory study of soldiers' attitudes toward a matched savings program in Korea. *Journal of Social Service Research, 44*(1), 30–37.

Kim, Y., Huang, J., Sherraden, M., & Clancy, M. (2017). Child development accounts, parental savings, and parental educational expectations: A path model. *Children and Youth Services Review, 79*(8), 20–28.

Lee, S. (2016). Performance and future directions of Seoul child development accounts. *Seoul Welfare Foundation Policy Report 2016-34*. Seoul: Seoul Welfare Foundation.

Nam, Y., & Han, C.-K. (2010). A new approach to promote economic independence among at-risk children: Child Development Accounts (CDAs) in Korea. *Children and Youth Services Review, 32*(11), 1548–1554.

Nho, C. R., Park, E. H., & McCarthy, M. L. (2017). Case studies of successful transition from out-of-home placement to young adulthood in Korea. *Children and Youth Services Review, 79*, 315–324.

Schreiner, M., Sherraden, M., Clancy, M., Johnson, L., Curley, J., Grinstein-Weiss, ... Beverly, S. (2001). *Savings and asset accumulation in individual development accounts*. St. Louis: Center for Social Development, George Warren Brown School of Social Work.

Sherraden, M. (1991). *Assets and the poor: A new American welfare policy*. New York, NY: M.E. Sharpe.

Sherraden, M. (2016, November 28). Asset building as policy innovation: Universal child development accounts. *Keynote Speech in Self-Sufficiency Welfare International Forum*. Seoul: Central Self-Sufficiency Foundation.

Ssewamala, F. M., Han, C.-K., & Neilands, T. (2009). Asset ownership and health and mental health functioning among AIDS-orphaned adolescents: Findings from a randomized clinical trial in rural Uganda. *Social Science & Medicine, 69*(2), 191–198.

Ssewamala, F. M., Han, C.-K., Neilands, T., Ismayilova, L., & Sperber, E. (2010). Effects of economic assets on sexual risk-taking intentions among orphaned adolescents in Uganda. *American Journal of Public Health, 100*(3), 483–488.

Yadama, G., & Sherraden, M. (1996). Effects of assets on attitudes and behaviors: Advance test of a social policy proposal. *Social Work Research, 20*(1), 3–11.

Yeo, Y. (2018). The current condition and policy issues of child poverty in Korea. *Health and Welfare Forum, 259*, 25–39.

Breaking the cycle: an asset-based family intervention for poverty alleviation in China

Suo Deng

ABSTRACT

Limited attention is given to how the poverty alleviation benefits children's development and breaking the transmission of intergenerational poverty in China. Based on two pilot programmes, *Chunyu* and *Qianshou*, in Shan'xi province, this study presents the potential effects of an asset-based family intervention that incorporates Child Development Accounts (CDAs) and parental support services on children and families. This study finds that the implementation of the programmes has positive financial and nonfinancial benefits for children and their families. The CDAs may serve as a key mechanism to integrate and strengthen the effect of asset building and parental involvement.

Introduction

China's rapid economic growth since the late 1970s enabled more than 700 million people to rise above the national poverty line, contributing to over 70% of the poverty reduced across the world (United Nation Development Programme, 2016). However, the dramatic socio-economic transition complicates the issue of poverty in China. The trickle-down effect of the initial natural economic growth has gradually weakened (Wang, Xu, & Shang, 2014), deepening the structural factors of poverty – namely, inequality and intergenerational poverty transmission. Addressing these issues requires sustained antipoverty measures and a strengthened social welfare system.

At the 18th National Congress of the Communist Party of China (CPC) in 2012, the Chinese government launched a new poverty alleviation plan in attempt to eradicate rural poverty and build an all-round moderately prosperous society by 2020. Featuring precise and targeted measures, the plan's primary goal is to ensure all of China's poor have enough to eat and wear, and receive adequate education, health services and housing. It emphasises the household as the unit of action, highlighting the importance of accurate poverty identification, appropriate project arrangement and accurate implementation to ensure that assistance reaches poverty-stricken households (Xinhuanet, 2016). Since 2013, this poverty alleviation plan has become the top policy priority at all levels of government, particularly in the west and in remote areas where poverty is critical.

Though the implementation of China's poverty alleviation plan has made great impacts, its sustainability has attracted increasing attention. The plan in many places largely follows the conventional understanding that poverty is merely a lack of income and basic living security, rather than the poor's capabilities for long-term development. Moreover, it is mostly adult-centred and gives limited attention to child development in poor families. China's current poverty alleviation plan does not adequately bridge the gap between vulnerable children in poor and non-poor households.

This qualitative study is based on two pilot programmes that incorporates Child Development Accounts (CDAs) and parental support services on children and families – *Chunyu* and *Qianshou* – implemented in Shan'xi province of China. It investigates the impact of these two asset-based family interventions on participating children and their families. The study begins by offering some background information about childhood vulnerability to poverty, parental practice and asset-building policy. The study's methods are reviewed before its findings are presented and discussed. It concludes with an exploration of how integrated CDA programmes can benefit China's poverty alleviation plan.

Background

This section provides context by reviewing the literature on intergenerational poverty and its relationship to childhood vulnerability and parental practice, asset-building policies across the globe and China's current research on asset-building policy to address intergenerational poverty.

Asset-based social policy and childhood poverty

Poverty and its relationship with social policy have undergone a paradigm shift since the mid-twentieth century. Though the traditional perspective of poverty focuses on deprivation of material goods in maintaining a basic living, the new consensus is oriented towards inequality and the poor's lack of capability to achieve meaningful development (Sen, 1999). Poverty is therefore viewed not as a static situation but as a dynamic process associated with vulnerability or poverty risks over a long period of time. A growing body of research has discovered the transmission of dynamic and chronic poverty across generations (Harper, Marcus, & Moore, 2003; Rank & Hirschl, 1999). In this regard, many countries have prioritised the strategies of investing in children to mitigate their vulnerability to break the intergenerational cycle of poverty (Midgley & Conley, 2010).

Poverty begins at home, during childhood. Childhood vulnerability is an important predictor of intergenerational poverty. Children from disadvantaged families lag significantly behind those from the advantaged ones in various development outcomes (e.g. academic scores, post-secondary education enrolment) (Lareau, 2003). Parental practice is a crucial factor of child development (Heckman, 2011). The differences between wealthy and poor families in parenting practice predict diverging destinies of children (Kalil, 2015).

Household asset holding may interplay with parenting practices in affecting children's development outcomes. Asset-based social policy approaches provide an insightful perspective on this. As noted by Sherraden (1991), *income* refers to the flow of resources, and is usually used for consumption of goods and services in a short time. In contrast, *assets* are the stock of wealth that can be used for cushioning people's income loss, education or business investment, or other activities towards developmental goals. The asset-based approach shifts away from needs-focused welfare, and moves forward to capacity building and development (Schreiner & Sherraden, 2007).

Asset accumulation not only creates economic opportunities, but also has positive socio-psychological effects on individuals and families (Paxton, 2001). Strong evidence exists on the impact of household asset holding on parenting, including parental expectation and investment towards the child's education (Kim & Sherraden, 2011; Yeung & Conley, 2008; Zhan & Sherraden, 2011). In particular, asset accumulation may motivate parents to invest in children, improve parenting behaviour and ultimately benefit children's development (Yeung & Conley, 2008). On the other hand, parental involvement, especially through parent–child communication and the transmission of parental educational expectations, may mediate the effect of asset accumulation, which in turn positively affects children's academic achievement and social–emotional development (Elliott III, 2009; Harkness & Newman, 2003; Zhan & Sherraden, 2011).

CDAs as an example of asset-based social policy

Inspired by asset-based theory, CDAs – savings or investment accounts for children with the purpose of developmental goals such as post-secondary education, home-ownership and career training – have been implemented in various countries worldwide (Loke & Sherraden, 2009; Sherraden et al., 2018a). Research demonstrates CDAs' positive impacts on the development of children and family as a whole (Clancy, Beverly, Sherraden, & Huang, 2016; Sherraden et al., 2018b).

The CDA intervention is based on the institutional theory of saving. It argues that people, particularly low-income people, require institutional support to accumulate and hold assets, and thereby build capability to combat poverty (Sherraden et al., 2018a). The CDA intervention has a positive impact on both children and families. Studies based on the SEED OK programme in the United States show that CDAs increase parental involvement in children and reduce the negative impact of family vulnerability on children's social and emotional development (Huang, Sherraden, Kim, & Clancy, 2014; Kim, Huang, Sherraden, & Clancy, 2017). In Uganda, for example, the CDA programme introduced a strong multidimensional development component to reduce family breakdown and provide effective and suitable care for vulnerable children (Curley, Ssewamala, Nabunya, Ilic, & Han, 2016).

In line with the asset-based framework, a growing body of research has investigated the effect of household asset holding on the development of children and youth in China (Deng, Sherraden, Huang, & Jin, 2013; Deng & Meng, 2013). Research calls for more progressive asset policy to address the challenges of poverty and long-term development of vulnerable children. Nonetheless, there has been limited research in testing the effect of CDA interventions in China's socio-cultural contexts. Less discussion involves connecting the CDA programme with more comprehensive poverty alleviation strategies to address intergenerational poverty transmission.

A national CDA policy could have important benefits for poverty alleviation in China. It could address intergenerational poverty transmission by not only providing short-term welfare services, but also enabling children to build assets to achieve life-long development goals. Though China currently has no established national CDA policy, two pilot CDA programmes, *Chunyu* and *Qianshou*, have been launched through collaboration bewteen the local government and non-profit organizations in Shan'xi Province. This study investigates the effect of these asset-based family interventions on China's socio-cultural context.

Methodology

This section reviews the programme design of the two CDA programmes, their demographic characteristics and this study's data collection.

Programme design

Both programmes in this study target vulnerable children and families in rural areas, aiming to promote their asset and capacity building. The *Chunyu* programme was implemented in a state-designated poverty county, Baishui of Shan'xi Province. With informed consent, a total of 10 children aged 12–16 years whose parents were having disabilities were identified to participate in this 4-year programme (2017–2021). In the participant selection process, *Chunyu* programme administrators considered potential participants' household economic situation, age of the child and the caregiver's disability status – as children of parents with disabilities are often among the most vulnerable in rural China. *Chunyu* consists of three intervention components: CDAs, financial education and parenting support. Parents or caregivers agreed to open a CDA in the child's name to help them accumulate assets for educational development. The child and family save in the account and the agency provides one-to-one monthly matches ranging from RMB 50 ($7.29 USD) to RMB 100 ($14.57 USD) with a cap of RMB 100. Accountholders can access the savings in the accounts after 1 year for children's educational purposes such as tuition, after-school tutoring and study tours. In addition, *Chunyu* offers children 2-hour financial education classes every month, focusing on basic knowledge of saving, loan and financial planning for future development. It also provides parents or caregivers programme information and updates on their children's performance through a social medial platform, Wechat. Parents are also invited to attend two 2-hour parenting workshops per year together with their children.

Qianshou was a 6-month programme (October, 2016–March, 2017) implemented in a rehabilitation service centre in Xi'an city of Shan'xi Province. Ten children and their parents or caregivers participated. Families were identified based on their economic situation and household registration status. Parents or caregivers, with informed consent, agreed to open CDAs for their children. Programme administrators provided an initial deposit of RMB 1500 ($219 USD) to each account to encourage continuous savings. Families could receive a one-to-one match for their monthly savings up to RMB 50 ($7.29 USD). In exchange for the matched deposits, parents or caregivers were required to carry out rehabilitation training for their children at home. *Qianshou* provided financial education workshops for parents or caregivers on money manage-ment and financial planning. The programme also offered monthly parenting classes on how to take care of children with developmental disabilities.

Demographic characteristics of participants

For the *Chunyu* programme, of the ten children participants, six were girls and four were boys. The age range was 13–15 years old, with the average being 14.2. All children were in middle school when they were involved in the programme. There exists a large variation in their family living arrangements. Four children often live with only one parent. Among them, the parents of two children divorced, and the fathers of the other two children-worked in the city for most of the year. In addition, three other children families can be considered skip-generational, as both of their parents often work in cities. All children participants were from low-income households, among which three were identified as poor, according to the official poverty line of RMB 3,015 ($443 USD) per capita.

In the *Qianshou* programme, the children participants consist of six boys and four girls, aged an average of 3.8 years. All participants were eligible for the government rehabilitation assistance programme for children with developmental disabilities younger than 6 years old. Though only one family is defined as income poor, all other families owed large amounts of debt from health care expenditure of their disabled children.

Data collection

For both programmes, the author serves as an external consultant and evaluator, and was involved in every stage of programme design and operation. Given the preliminary nature of the programme and the research, a qualitative approach was undertaken for a deep understanding of the project implementation process and experience of parti-cipants. A participatory approach was adopted for evaluation for more detailed reflec-tion of the experiences, expressions and views of project participants and other stakeholders.

Focus Group Discussions and in-depth interviews were conducted with participating children and their caregivers, as well as case managers and the agency director. Other data sources were obtained from case records, document review and observation of activities. With the agreement of the participants, some interviews were audio taped and transcribed afterward. All qualitative data, including transcripts, ethnographic notes and bibliographic data, were systematically coded for subsequent analysis. The author deploys a grounded theory method for data analysis (Strauss, 1987). As a result, discourses concerning participants' feelings are captured and interpreted, and the out-comes, effects and challenges of the programme are tentatively evaluated.

Findings

The implementation of the programmes has shown some positive results on participat-ing children and their families. The following section elaborates the two main findings:

the CDA programmes had (1) financial benefits for children and families, and (2) nonfinancial benefits for children and families.

Financial benefits for children and families

Through opening and managing CDAs and taking the financial education training, participants in both programmes gained better access to mainstream financial products and increased their financial literacy. As a result, participants strengthened their financial knowledge, enabling them to build assets for human development.

Many *Chunyu* participants lived in a state of asset deprivation, lacking access and the basic means to build assets for their family's economic development (e.g. secured savings, loans). Moreover, China's current adult-centred poverty alleviation plan did not effectively mitigate their vulnerability, leaving many to face serious economic insecurity in terms of education and health care. According to the interviews with participants, education and health care are the top of household expenditures. Though the compulsory education law covers tuition and fees for children at primary or middle schools, other school-related expenses such as food, after-school tutoring and transportation remain a relative high burden for them. The CDA component of *Chunyu* assisted participating families in managing their finances and securing investment in their children's education.

For families with children with developmental disabilities, household economic circumstances tended to be even more complicated. This is the key issue that the *Qianshou* programme attempts to address. Early rehabilitation is enormously expensive. Aside from the basic health care schemes, poor families with disabled children do not have enough accumulated assets to buffer the economic pressure of rehabilitation. In fact, the average debts for the participating families of the programme were more than 50,000 RMB ($7276 USD). Therefore, the need for CDA programmes such as *Qianshou* is high.

In interviews, parents of children in both *Chunyu* and *Qianshou* expressed that they had never thought of opening an account for their children before. One major reason is that it is unusual to open a banking account in a child's name with local financial institutions. Though mainstream banking for children is legal in China, many institutional barriers exist in practice that exclude them. For example, in Baishui County, local banks require the child's birth certificate and identification card to process the account opening application. However, most rural parents do not apply for these documents for their children at birth, opting instead to handle it when their children go to work. In addition, local financial institutions usually charge annual fees on accounts with a low balance, which makes account opening unattractive for poor families.

By opening CDAs for children, both programmes helped children gain the access to banks for the first time, granting the opportunity to save and plan for the future. In an interview, an 11-year-old boy, MGY,[1] in the first year of middle school shared his learning experience in the programme after 1 year:

> After joining in the programme, I had the opportunity to go to the bank with my mom to open my own bank account. It was my first time going to a bank. I learned how to deposit money and set a password at the counter. My mom gives me RMB10 every week for snacks and stationaries, and I can save some in my account. For example, if I have RMB30, I will leave RMB10 for later use, RMB5 for saving and the rest for current use.

Both programmes provide regular financial education workshops for children and caregivers. The workshops deliver basic financial knowledge, including saving and withdrawing procedures, how to set an appropriate saving goal that aligns with developmental needs, and how to avoid online financial fraud. A programme case manager mentioned that children could learn and practice financial-related knowledge through these workshops, but have almost no chance from their formal school education. She noticed that children actually had great interest in learning financial knowledge because it is practical and useful.

In addition to the children gaining financial knowledge and skills, their parents or caregivers also benefited from attending workshops and managing the accounts. One example is the case of ZXF, the father of a 3-year-old girl with cerebral palsy in the *Qianshou* programme. ZXF had always been anxious about his daughter's rehabilitation. He had spent much money seeking and experimenting folk prescriptions and owed a large amount of debt. Since joining *Qianshou*, he had become more aware of his family's economic situation. He was more willing to listen to other people's suggestions and learn to spend more rationally and wisely, trying to balance the expenditure on his child's health care and other family living expenses.

A mother of a 6-year-old girl also talked about how the CDA changed her thinking and behaviour about saving and spending:

> Although a 100 RMB deposit each month does not seem a large amount of money, accumulation of one year's savings can really help to solve some bigger problems. I think this plan pushes me to think of my spending and the family's financial life over time. The savings are required to be used for children's education and rehabilitation, not for eating or clothing. This is good to plan my child's health care and other expenditures now and in the future.

Participants in both programmes had actively engaged in financial asset building for children's education and health care. The *Chunyu* programme offered a 1:1 matching deposit for any amount of saving from RMB 50 to the cap of RMB100, and all participants except one chose the maximum amount of saving after 5 months. One and half years later, the total amount of savings reached RMB 20,100, with nine participants holding RMB 1800 respectively and one RMB 900 in the CDAs.

The children participants were relatively younger in the *Qianshou* programme. Parents or caregivers therefore took the main responsibility to open and manage CDAs. The parents or caregivers understood that the goal of the CDA was to save money to meet the development needs of children. According to the case manager, all caregivers expressed that they would continue to save for their children even after the programme ended.

The above qualitative evidence suggests that CDAs may become a critical vehicle to nurture and increase the family's financial awareness, helping them plan family spending on children's development and other consumption items. Children were able to access financial products in early ages and likely established a good saving habit.

Children from poor households are often excluded from the institutional opportunity to accumulate financial assets and lack of financial literacy (Sherraden, 2013). The CDA and financial education components in *Chunyu* provide them with an opportunity to engage in and benefit from the asset-building process. In *Qianshou*, the saving goals were more concrete and designed to be achieved in a shorter term because participants faced greater economic burdens due to their children's disability status. Both programmes offered financial benefits for participants.

Nonfinancial benefits for children and families

Participating in either *Chunyu* or *Qianshou* also offers nonfinancial benefits. Participating children and their parents or caregivers demonstrate stronger future orientation and improved parent–child interactions. These effects result from a mutual enhancement of asset-building and parental support strategies.

The CDAs enable a shift in the parents' cognitive focus from daily stressors to future development. The families participating in the CDA programmes had long been struggling with multiple challenges, including health problems, unemployment, care for children with disabilities and debt. Entangled with short-term livelihood needs, parents and caregivers tend to concentrate on the problems rather than the potential advantages of their families (Mani, Mullainathan, Shafir, & Zhao, 2013). The CDA programmes provided opportunities for families to make decisions for their children's future.

In addition to building assets, CDAs also change attitudes towards future development, such as educational expectations. Children and parents often have different educational expectations. The baseline assessment in *Chunyu* programme found that parents had high educational expectations for their children, but many children tended to view their educational future as very gloomy. The preliminary evaluation shows that participation in the project has greatly improved children's confidence in future development. By combining asset-building and parental support services, the CDA programmes contribute to these positive changes by offering opportunities to develop financial knowledge and skills. In addition, the intervention targeted parent–child interaction to create opportunities for two generations to communicate with and ultimately understand each other.

In the *Chunyu* programme, most parents noticed and were excited about the changes in their children's attitudes and behaviours. The programme case manager indicated that participating children could better understand some abstract concepts such as life goals and future planning:

> Usually when you teach children about future development, they cannot understand the contents and tend to have no interest. But if they have knowledge about saving, they often could understand that it is related to their future development. This way of learning therefore is a very specific and useful method. From my understanding, the CDA programme could help the children form good morality and behaviour, which will definitely benefit their school study and future education.

Intergenerational communication benefits both children and parents/caregivers by enhancing their mutual understanding and forming positive attitudes towards each other. Both programmes emphasise the importance of more parental involvement in children's education and health care. Indeed, by gaining financial knowledge, children can better understand their parents' difficulties in earning a living. On the other hand, parents have the chance to see and think about their children's future and life goals. An interview with one parent of a boy aged 14 years old, LS, who was enrolled in *Chunyu* reflected this point:

> We don't have much money as parents, but we still give our kid some pocket money every week, as he needs to buy necessities at school. He also receives red packets in the lunar New Year. Since participation in the programme, he has learned to save money. Last month he did deposit some money in his CDA. I became more aware of his future and often discuss with him about the future plan, such as 'what you want to do if you are not able to enter college', 'what do you really like to be when you grow up', 'what you can do', etc. I think he can understand more about these questions now.

A mother of the child aged 13 years from *Chunyu* shared her experience:

> I think that the CDA programme helps to develop children's financial planning awareness and also is good for developing a self-management habit. It teaches children the sense of valuing, not only valuing the money but more importantly valuing other people including his parents. Before, when we bought something for him, he was not respectful. After joining the programme, he has learned to save money. Now when he wants to buy something, he will think first if it is really necessary. He learned how to value something. I think this is the biggest change for my child.

The *Qianshou* programme had more requirements for parents' or caregivers' involvement in rehabilitation training at home for their disabled children. Taking care of a child with disabilities is difficult, especially for low-income families. The asset-based family intervention with a CDA component helped build family capability in the process of a child's rehabilitation. It enabled parents or caregivers to think beyond daily life difficulties and plan their child's future development.

In *Qianshou*, parents and caregivers received more intensive parenting support services, including workshops on how to provide quality caregiving to a child with cerebral palsy and how to budget the children's health care expenditure. The parenting support services taught and reinforced basic parenting skills, such as how to communicate effectively with children. In the parenting workshops, peer family groups formed an informal network through which they could support each other on parenting and financial decision-making.

The existing research has demonstrated that parents from the disadvantaged families, compared with their counterparts from advantaged ones, often do not have future-oriented planning for their children (Kalil, 2015). Related research in behavioural economics reveals the impact of parents' financial stress on children. Parents who must devote the majority of their cognitive attention to balancing the daily family expenses leave little room to follow through on decisions that can affect their children's future development (Mani et al., 2013). Such households trapped in the cycle of poverty often face asset constraints, meaning they lack adequate assets to meet their development needs beyond current consumption. Nonetheless, conventional family service programmes targeting parental behaviour change have been deemed ineffective due to failure in motivating family asset building and parental involvement in a sustainable way (Wagner, Spiker, & Linn, 2002). Built on the vehicle of CDAs, the *Chunyu* and *Qianshou* aim to develop family capabilities through monitoring the saving and asset accumulation process. The establishment of CDAs may motivate parents to invest in their children. Furthermore, by incorporating the component of goal-directed parenting support services, the two programmes would reinforce the association between asset building and the development of the whole family.

Discussion

China's new poverty alleviation plan places great emphasis on adapting targeted measures to lift individuals and families out of poverty. The asset-based policy approach can provide important insights for the outcome and sustainability of poverty alleviation. By focusing on breaking the cycle of intergenerational poverty transmission, this qualitative study based on two small-scale programmes aims to examine the potential effects of the asset-based family intervention that incorporates CDAs and parental support services on vulnerable children and families. Preliminary evidence provides evidence that the implementation of the programmes has positive financial and non-financial benefits for children and the family.

First, by opening CDAs, children and parents/caregivers gained greater access to financial products that benefit their future development. They had opportunities to engage in the whole process of accumulating financial assets including opening, managing and saving in an account. In the meantime, they acquired relevant knowledge and skills of asset accumulation through attending regular financial educational trainings. Furthermore, participating children and parents/caregivers showed positive changes in developing future orientation and improving parent–child interactions.

From the participatory evaluation of the project implementation process including in-depth interviews with participants, this paper argues that there is a positive correlation between asset building and family support interventions. As an important mechanism, CDAs play a key role in promoting or maximising the interactive effects of asset building and parental involvement.

Asset-based family interventions, such as CDAs, have great implications for China's poverty alleviation plan. Though the plan is greatly beneficial to extremely poor households, the vulnerability of many of these families will likely pull them back into poverty, given the nature of intergenerational poverty. Their asset constraints may lead to deprivation of children's development opportunities, which are often neglected or sacrificed when families lack adequate economic resources. Parental practice plays a critical meditating role between household economic circumstance and child development outcome. However, the current parenting programmes in China's poverty alleviation plan do not go far enough to produce sustained effects on children. Therefore, implementing a national CDA policy could become an important way to strengthen China's poverty alleviation plan. It could address intergenerational poverty transmission by not only providing short-term welfare services, but also enabling children to build assets to achieve life-long development goals.

Study limitations

The limitations of this study should be noted. First, the two programmes are relatively small in scale, and their evaluation is still preliminary. The two projects also have some comparability problems. Though both have core elements of a CDA intervention, there are significant differences in project design, project duration and participants; therefore, the conclusions drawn should be interpreted carefully. Second, though the qualitative approach of this study can help describe the implementation process of the project and the participants' feelings, the intervention effect calls for more rigorous experimental design methods to verify. Continuous evaluation of the project would provide more supplementary information. It is expected that future CDA projects can be expanded to provide more rigorous evaluation and research data information.

Conclusion

After 40 years of reform and opening up, China's poverty problem and its characteristics have undergone significant changes. The issue of poverty has increasingly been linked to inequality and vulnerability resulting from the dramatic socioeconomic transition of recent decades. The changes call for more innovative social policies and a strengthened social service system. Though income-based poverty alleviation strategies are still fundamental, changing social risks require more progressive social policy interventions to promote asset building of poor individuals and families to achieve long-term social protection (Deng et al., 2013). The asset-based family interventions examined in this study are expected to not simply have positive effects on children, but also help the whole family build capabilities through promoting the family's asset accumulation and positive parenting practices. The implementation of these two programmes, though still ongoing, has important implications for China's poverty alleviation strategies in the new era of socioeconomic development.

Note

1. We use initials of the interviewee's name for anonymity (same as below).

Disclosure statement

No potential conflict of interest was reported by the author.

References

Clancy, M. M., Beverly, S. G., Sherraden, M., & Huang, J. (2016). Testing universal child development accounts: Financial impacts in a large social experiment. *Social Service Review*, *90*(4), 683–708.

Curley, J., Ssewamala, F. M., Nabunya, P., Ilic, V., & Han, C.-K. (2016). Child development accounts (CDAs): An asset-building strategy to empower girls in Uganda. *Social Work*, *59*(1), 18–31.

Deng, S. & Meng, Y. (2013). Financial access and economic participation of youth with disabilities in China: An exploratory study. *China Journal of Social Work*, *6*(2), 177–189.

Deng, S., Sherraden, M., Huang, J., & Jin, M. (2013). Asset opportunity for the poor: An asset-based policy agenda towards inclusive growth in China. *China Journal of Social Work*, *6*(1), 40–51.

Elliott, W., III. (2009). Children's college aspirations and expectations: The potential role of children's development accounts (CDAs). *Children and Youth Services Review*, *31*(2), 274–283.

Harkness, J. M., & Newman, S. (2003). The effects of homeownership on children: The role of neighborhood characteristics and family income. *Economic Policy Review*, *9*(2), 87–107.

Harper, C., Marcus, R., & Moore, K. (2003). Enduring poverty and the conditions of childhood: Lifecourse and intergenerational poverty transmissions. *World Development*, *31*(3), 535–554.

Heckman, J. (2011). *The American family in black and white: A post-racial strategy for improving skills to promote equality* (National Bureau of economic research working paper No. 16841). Cambridge, MA: National Bureau of Economic Research.

Huang, J., Sherraden, M., Kim, Y., & Clancy, M. (2014). Effects of child development accounts on early social-emotional development: An experimental test. *JAMA Pediatrics*, *168*(3), 265–271.

Kalil, A. (2015). Inequality begins at home: The role of parenting in the diverging destinies of rich and poor children. In P. R. Amato, A. Booth, S. M. McHale, & J. V. Hook (Eds.), *Families in an era of increasing inequality: Diverging destinies* (pp. 63–82). New York, NY: Springer.

Kim, Y., Huang, J., Sherraden, M., & Clancy, M. (2017). Child development accounts, parental savings, and parental educational expectations: A path model. *Children and Youth Services Review*, *79*, 20–28.

Kim, Y., & Sherraden, M. (2011). Do parental assets matter for children's educational outcomes? Evidence from mediation tests. *Children and Youth Services Review*, *33*(6), 969–979.

Lareau, A. (2003). *Unequal childhoods: Class, race, and family life*. Berkeley, CA: University of Califonia Press.

Loke, V., & Sherraden, M. (2009). Building assets from birth: A global comparison of child development account policies. *International Journal of Social Welfare*, *18*, 119–129.

Mani, A., Mullainathan, S., Shafir, E., & Zhao, J. (2013). Poverty impedes cognitive function. *Science*, *30*, 976–980.

Midgley, J., & Conley, A. (2010). *Social work and social development: Theories and skills for developmental social work*. Cambridge: Oxford University Press.

Paxton, W. (2001). The asset-effect: An overview. In J. Bynner & W. Paxton (Eds.), *The asset-effect* (pp. 1–17). London, UK: Institute for Public Policy Research.

Rank, M. R., & Hirschl, T. A. (1999). The economic risk of childhood in America: Estimating the probability of poverty across the formative years. *Journal of Marriage and the Family*, *61* (November), 1058–1067.

Schreiner, M., & Sherraden, M. (2007). *Can the poor save? Savings and asset building in individual development accounts*. New Brunswick, NJ: Transaction.

Sen, A. K. (1999). *Commodities and capabilities*. Oxford, UK: Oxford University Press.

Sherraden, M. (1991). *Assets and the poor: A new American welfare policy*. Armonk, New York: M. E. Sharpe, Inc.

Sherraden, M. (2013). Building blocks of financial capability. In M. S. Sherraden & J. C. Curley (Eds.), *Financial capability and asset building: Research, education, policy, and practice* (pp.3–43). New York, NY: Oxford University Press.

Sherraden, M., Cheng, L.-C., Ssewamala, F. M., Kim, Y., Loke, V., Zou, L., ... Han, C.-K. (2018a). In C. Franklin et al. (Eds.), International child development accounts. *Encyclopedia of Social Work*. doi:10.1093/acrefore/9780199975839.013.1261.

Sherraden, M., Clancy, M., Nam, Y., Huang, J., Kim, Y., Beverly, S. G., ... Purnell, J. Q. (2018b). Universal and progressive child development accounts: A policy innovation to reduce educational disparity. *Urban Education, 53*(6), 806–833.

Strauss, A. L. (1987). *Qualitative analysis for social scientists*. New York, NY: Cambridge University Press.

United Nations Development Programme. (2016). China human development report. Retrieved from http://www.cn.undp.org/content/china/en/home/library/human_development/china-human-development-report-2016.html

Wagner, M., Spiker, D., & Linn, M. (2002). The effectiveness of the parents as teachers program with low-income parents and children. *Topics in Early Childhood Special Education, 22*, 67–81.

Wang, X., Xu, L., & Shang, X. (2014). China's pro-poor growth: Measurement and implications. *Journal of Social Service Research, 40*(1), 520–529.

Xinhuanet. (2016). China's cabinet issues five-year plan for poverty alleviation. *Retrieved November, 12*, 2017.

Yeung, W. J., & Conley, D. (2008). Black-white achievement gap and family wealth. *Child Development, 79*(2), 303–324.

Zhan, M., & Sherraden, M. (2011). Assets and liabilities, educational expectations, and children's college degree attainment. *Children and Youth Services Review, 33*(6), 846–854.

Policy models for child development accounts: vision, potential, strategies

Jin Huang, Michael Sherraden and Li Zou

In this book, we explore the global impact of child development accounts (CDAs). CDAs are a social policy innovation to begin universal, progressive, and potentially lifelong asset building (Sherraden, 1991). The larger purposes of CDAs are social inclusion, social justice, and social development.

The chapters in this book present CDA policy development and research in seven different countries and regions, including several examples from the Asia-Pacific area. This is the first book to examine this policy innovation in the global context. These examples show broad and growing interest in CDAs and expansion of asset-based social policies.

This conclusion summarizes the themes found throughout the book. It discusses the overall vision of CDAs and asset building, reviews the financial impacts of CDAs, explores the social development impacts of CDAs, and provides an outline for stable and efficient CDA policy design. It concludes with some recommendations for future research, policy, and practice.

A vision of CDAs and asset building

The countries that have implemented CDAs vary widely by geographic location, population size, culture and history, social and economic development, political institutions, and social welfare policy design. However, in a globalized, information-era economy, they all share the challenge of promoting social development. When considering how to meet this challenge, the questions are large: How can a society effectively and efficiently invest in all of its citizens to maximize their potential and opportunities? How can a society enable individuals and families to develop? How can a society promote inclusive economic growth? And how can a society achieve social well-being?

These questions go beyond the vision of traditional social programs, which are aimed at satisfying basic needs and maintaining a minimum level of consumption security. Goals of social inclusion, social justice, and social development can only be accomplished through purposeful *social development* strategies and *institution building*. In contrast, individual development strategies that primarily focus on "behavioral" approaches risk reinforcing the extreme economic inequality now present in many countries.

Social development takes a progressive view of the roles social policies can play in building a society, economy, and polity. The focus is not simply on maintenance, but also on improving capacities of individuals, families, and communities to reach their potential and add value to the larger society. Social development embodies a more accurate under-standing of social policies in "mixed economies." Because all economies are to some extent mixed, with blurred boundaries between social and economic policies, smart policy design recognizes this joint development challenge—social and economic—rather than assuming that one is a prerequisite or a drain on the other.

The challenge lies in identifying policy innovations and institutional arrangements that generate positive social and economic development together. The CDA policy studies in this book represent important real world examples of these efforts. Moreover, they are theoretically sound, logically feasible, purposeful, and evidence-supported. A solid foun-dation has been established from previous policy research (e.g., Sherraden et al., 2018), and the studies in this book strengthen that foundation.

Financial impacts of CDAs

In the larger picture, CDAs can be a policy platform that connects financial investment with social development in a highly financialized society. Consistent with previous research (Beverly et al., 2015; Clancy et al., 2016; Huang et al., 2015; Lewis et al., 2017; Nam et al., 2013), studies in the book suggest positive financial outcomes of CDAs for children and families, including those on account holding, asset accumulation, financial incentives and awards, and financial investment strategies.

For example, with an automatic enrollment mechanism, Post-Secondary Educational Accounts in Singapore (Part I Chapter 1) and SEED OK in the United States (Part I Chap-ter 3) successfully create an almost 100% account holding rate. Even requiring participant action, 69% of Israeli households eligible for the Save for Every Child Program (Part I Chapter 2) have made positive decisions on fund management in the first 5 months. In Taiwan, approximately 45% of eligible families opened CDAs and three-quarters of accountholders made family contributions in the first year (Chapter 4). Table C.1 sum-marizes the main CDA policy features across countries that generate positive financial impacts for children and families.

Table C.1 demonstrates how CDA policy creates new opportunities and financial tools for societies to invest in all children, universally. As discussed in the introductory chapter, universality (i.e., including all children in each country) should be a central goal of CDAs. Automatic enrollment for all children is the most efficient way to achieve universal CDAs. Through universality, CDAs become a structured institution and a stable infrastructure for social investment, maximizing impacts of both public and private resources. Because univer-sal CDAs provide savings and investment accounts for all children, they have the potential to include financially excluded children and families in the mainstream financial system.

We emphasize that *CDAs are much more than a bunch of savings accounts* resulting from individual behaviors. CDAs are an *institutional structure* for development of all children. In CDAs, to a large extent, the structure itself is doing the "behaving" in building assets. In this sense, CDAs can thought of as a public utility or a public good. Just as plumbing does much of the "behaving" in getting water to our houses, and public roads do much of the "behaving" in getting us from here to there, CDAs are a public policy that structures and supports the building of assets for all children.

Table C.1. CDA Policy Features and Financial Impacts.

Study	Account Holding	Asset Accumulation	Financial Investment
Singapore	• Automatically opened Edusave accounts • Opt-in SCDAs • Automatically opened PSEAs • Automatically opened Medisave accounts	• First-step funds provided by the government • Additional top-up funds from the government • Family contributions	• Guaranteed interested rate
Israel	• Automatically opened SECP accounts	• Monthly deposits from the government • Family contributions	• Bank account interest • Low-risk investment • Medium-risk investment • High-risk investment
United States	• Automatically opened state-owned college savings accounts • Opt-in individual-owned college savings accounts	• Seed deposits provided by the CDA program • Savings match to family contributions • Family contributions	• A variety of investment options offered by the College Savings Plans
Taiwan	• Opt-in bank accounts	• Savings match to family contributions from the government • Family contributions	• Bank account interest
Uganda	• Opt-in bank accounts	• Savings match to family contributions from the government • Individual contributions	• Bank account interest
Korea	• Opt-in bank accounts	• Savings match to family contributions from the government • Individual contributions • Funds from social sponsors	• Bank account interest
Mainland China	• Opt-in bank accounts	• Savings match to family contributions from the government • Family contributions	• Bank account interest

Moreover, from the perspective of a financial capability framework (Sherraden, 2013), financial inclusion can be achieved through universal CDAs. If all individuals own CDAs, they are included in the mainstream financial services and can build knowledge and practice financial skills with this account. In addition, many CDA policies offer financial education and guidance to support sound financial decisions. In other words, not only assets are being built, but also the access, experience, knowledge, and capability to function financially.

Social development impacts of CDAs

Despite their financial benefits, CDAs are not a solely economic intervention. They purposefully link asset accumulation and financial investment to both short- and long-term social development outcomes. For example, research documents the ways in which CDAs (1) enable parents to maintain high expectations for their children's education (e.g., Kim et al., 2015); (2) improve parents' mental outlook (e.g., Huang, Sherraden, & Purnell,

2014); (3) support children's social–emotional development (e.g., Huang et al., 2014); and (4) improve educational outcomes (e.g., Huang et al., 2010).

The studies in this book support these findings through triangulation of data, strengthening the understanding of the social development impacts of CDAs. For example, SEED OK research in the United States (Part I Chapter 3) was the first study to report positive impacts of CDAs on parenting behaviors and parent–child interactions. Supported by qualitative evidence in previous research (Gray et al., 2012), CDAs create a new and constructive family engagement toward development, shared by both parents and children. Based on another experimental study, the Uganda research (Part II Chapter 2) offers strong evidence that CDAs improve academic performance and educational attainment for highly disadvantaged children. Qualitative research from Korea (Part II Chapter 3) and China (Part IIChapter 4), synthesizing research in the United States with that of other countries (Gray et al., 2012; Johnson et al., 2015), also finds that CDAs generate hope, shape expectations, and facilitate future planning.

Because CDAs are in the early implementation stages, little is yet known about long-term social development effects. However theoretical and empirical reasons exist to hypothesize that CDA assets will enable positive developmental achievements, including post-secondary education, health, home ownership, and other asset investments over the long term.

In the meantime, it is important to note that short-term positive effects of CDAs occur during a period when assets are accumulating and are not yet spent. Researchers typically connect social policy expenditures with positive effects; however, in asset-building policy, the first focus is accumulation rather than expenditure (Part I Chapter 3). Research finds *positive effects during accumulation* (Beverly et al., 2015; Clancy et al., 2016; Huang, Nam, & Sherraden, 2015; Lewis et al., 2017; Nam et al., 2013). Future additional positive effects—when CDA assets are used for education and other social development purposes—can be anticipated.

Another important policy point is that CDAs can readily merge with and support other important policies, such as education, job training, and health and behavior interventions. In the United States, it is not uncommon that CDAs integrate with a variety of social services provided by local community agencies (Huang et al., 2019). In this book, for example, the CDA intervention in Uganda (Chapter 6) offers mentorship and financial planning services in addition to the account. The CDA demonstration in China (Chapter 8) accommodates training lessons for parents of children with developmental disabilities. In the process, CDAs can multiply positive social-development outcomes.

A safe, stable, and efficient policy model for CDAs

Expanding CDAs and positive effects to all children, and making them long lasting, will require a safe, stable, and efficient policy model. The policy model is fundamental, yet most "policy research" does not address it. Instead, most policy research focuses on individual outcomes, without considering the details about how the policy is shaped and implemented. Such an approach does not provide adequate guidance on how to create a successful social innovation. Measuring and assessing safety, stability, efficiency, and other policy features is central to understanding a strong CDA policy model. Researchers at the Center for Social Development at Washington University in St. Louis have long considered the essential elements of a strong CDA policy model: universality, progressivity, and lifelong in nature.

From the outset, SEED OK tested a safe, efficient, and sustainable policy design, based on many years of testing asset-based policies. The thinking on policy design continues to be refined based on research data, policy experiences, and policy practice. To this end, the Center for Social Development suggests ten key design elements for safe, efficient, and sustainable CDAs at scale: (1) universal eligibility, (2) automatic enrollment, (3) at-birth start, (4) automatic initial deposits, (5) automatic progressive subsidy, (6) centralized savings plan, (7) investment growth potential, (8) targeted investment options, (9) restricted withdrawals, and (10) means-tested public benefit exclusions (Clancy & Beverly, 2017; Sherraden, Clancy, & Beverly, 2018).

These are straightforward, achievable goals based on real world policy conditions. Different policymakers may rank certain elements as higher priorities, but universal eligibility and automatic enrollment are foundational. Automatic features on enrollment, deposits, and subsidies are the most efficient elements to overcome socioeconomic and behavioral barriers among eligible families. A centralized savings plan—as in 401(k) plans, or the Federal Thrift Savings plan—ensures safety and stability of account services, and has the potential for large-scale applications. The final element on public benefit exclusions emphasizes that CDAs should not cause participants to become ineligible for public benefits.

Together, these design elements form a strong CDA policy model. This work has been generated mainly in the United States, particularly from the SEED OK experiment. Though the SEED OK experiment satisfies all of these elements, this does not mean it represents the perfect policy design. It is possible—even likely—that different economic and financial infrastructure conditions in different countries will determine how these design elements can best be implemented. However, based on the policy experiences and research presented in this book, we suggest that the ten key CDA design elements, in some form, can be applied globally.

In this regard, the studies in this book represent case studies of CDA policy models and features. Comparisons across these case studies may offer insights into building a CDA policy model. In Table C.2, we compare these case studies against the ten design elements. This comparison documents that CDA policies are (very understandably) different, adapted to social, economic, and political circumstances where they are implemented.

It also could be that CDA policies and programs may be at different developmental stages, all trending toward an ideal of fully inclusive and sustainable CDAs—but needless to say, this sort of ideal interpretation does not often reflect patterns and potential in the real world. The best we can hope for is that countries can and will learn from each other. The conference that generated the chapters in this book, and the book itself, provide an example of this exchange and learning.

Table C.2. Comparing CDA Policy Models: Ten Design Elements.

Design Element	Singapore	Israel	United States	Taiwan	Uganda	Korea	Mainland China
Universal eligibility	✓	✓	✓	×	×	×	×
Automatic enrollment	✓	✓	✓	×	×	×	×
At-birth start	✓	✓	✓	✓	×	×	×
Automatic initial deposits	✓	×	✓	×	×	×	×
Automatic progressive subsidy	×	×	✓	✓	✓	✓	✓
Centralized savings plan	✓	✓	✓	×	×	×	×
Investment growth potential	✓	✓	✓	✓	✓	✓	×
Targeted investment options	×	✓	✓	×	×	×	×
Restricted withdrawals	✓	✓	✓	✓	✓	✓	×
Means-tested public benefit exclusions	✓	✓	✓	✓	✓	✓	✓

Conclusion

After the CDA policy concept was proposed in the early 1990s, a variety of CDA policies and programs have been implemented around the world. Many small, less-documented CDA applications are not presented in this book, and other country-level discussions of CDAs are now almost common. Positive CDA impacts on families and children are documented, and successful policy design features are coming into focus. Since these chapters were written, CDA policy has continued to proliferate. For example, several U.S. states have enacted universal policies, Taiwan has implemented policy improvements, and mainland China and Azerbaijan are designing CDA demonstrations. Some countries have achieved safe, efficient, and sustainable CDA policy at large scale. However, stable and strong CDA policies are not yet widespread; there is still work to do. Further research and replication in more countries will be required.

Built on the current CDA implementation, demonstration, and research, how can we achieve the grand vision that every child on the earth might have an asset-building account? In traveling towards this vision, it will be important to hold fast to basic CDA principles as a lodestar in guiding policy. In this regard, full inclusion, automatic enrollment, and progressivity are at the forefront. Chapters in this book represent CDA examples at different policy development stages and in diverse nations.

If CDA policy becomes common at a national level, it will reach the largest populations possible. For this purpose, the key challenge of policymakers is to design and implement national CDAs following strong policy models. Several tasks are necessary to achieve this goal. More research will be required to understand how to design and implement strong CDA models, in addition to other core research questions, especially "What are the effects of CDAs?" and "How can we best support family asset building?"

Experiences and lessons from CDA implementation also offer practitioners a footing for bottom-up approaches to grow local CDA programs into a general social policy. In this regard, it may be helpful to build a global network among CDAs among policymakers, practitioners, and researchers to learn from each other and work toward high-level, large-scale CDA policies.

As always, the pathway will not be predictable, smooth, and easy. National CDA policy (or any asset-building policy) may encounter limitations in capacities of policy institutions, honesty of governments, and macroeconomic management. Long-term asset building always faces these challenges; but we have also seen that that these potential limitations can be overcome. In this regard, the example of Singapore (Part I Chapter 1) merits greater attention around the world than it has yet received.

The future also holds greater potential. With advancements in financial technology—perhaps including digital currencies—international CDAs, reaching across national boundaries, could create asset-building policy that serves all children globally. It is not inconceivable that international development banks could, over the next several decades, create life-long digital accounts for all newborns on the planet. *Technology will make global CDAs highly efficient and achievable.* To be sure, political and economic challenges, like the weather, will always be with us—but coping is possible. Principles to achieve strong CDA national policy models could be incorporated into international CDAs.

Taking this thinking a step further, international CDAs might bring developed and developing countries closer together, creating greater access, opportunity, social development, and economic stability globally. This ideal can never be fully achieved, but positive steps in this direction are worthwhile and very possible.

References

Beverly, S. G., Kim, Y., Sherraden, M., Nam, Y., & Clancy, M. (2015). Can Child Development Accounts be inclusive? Early evidence from a statewide experiment. *Children and Youth Services Review, 53*, 92–104.

Clancy, M. M., & Beverly, S. G. (2017). Statewide Child Development Account policies: Key design elements. St. Louis, MO: Center for Social Development, Washington University in St. Louis.

Clancy, M. M., Beverly, S. G., Sherraden, M., & Huang, J. (2016). Testing universal child development accounts: Financial effects in a large social experiment. *Social Service Review, 90*(4), 683–708.

Gray, K., Clancy, M., Sherraden, M. S., Wagner, K., Miller-Cribbs, J. (2012). Interviews with mothers of young children in the SEED for Oklahoma Kids College Savings Experiment (CSD Research Report 12-53). Center for Social Development, Washington University in St. Louis, St. Louis, MO. Retrieved March 21, 2014 from http://csd.wustl.edu/Publications/Documents/RP12-53.pdf

Huang, J., Beverly, S. G., Kim, Y., Clancy, M. M., & Sherraden, M. (2019). Exploring a model for integrating Child Development Accounts with social services for vulnerable families. *Journal of Consumer Affairs, 53*(3), 770–795.

Huang, J., Guo, B., Kim, Y., & Sherraden, M. (2010). Parental income, assets, borrowing constraints and children's post-secondary education. *Children and Youth Services Review, 32*(4), 585–594.

Huang, J., Nam, Y., Sherraden, M., & Clancy, M. (2015). Financial capability and asset accumulation for children's education: Evidence from an experiment of child development accounts. *Journal of Consumer Affairs, 49*(1), 127–155.

Huang, J., Sherraden, M., Kim, Y., & Clancy, M. (2014). Effects of Child Development Accounts on early social-emotional development: An experimental test. *JAMA pediatrics, 168*(3), 265–271.

Huang, J., Sherraden, M., & Purnell, J. Q. (2014). Impacts of Child Development Accounts on maternal depressive symptoms: Evidence from a randomized statewide policy experiment. *Social Science & Medicine, 112*, 30–38.

Johnson, L., Lee, Y., Ansong, D., Sherraden, M.S., Chowa, G., Ssewamala, F., Zou, L., Sherraden, M., . . . Saavedra, J. (2015). Youth savings patterns and performance in Colombia, Ghana, Kenya, and Nepal. St. Louis, MO: Center for Social Development, Washington University. Retrieved from https://openscholarship.wustl.edu/cgi/viewcontent.cgi?article=1762&context=csd_research

Kim, Y., Sherraden, M., Huang, J., & Clancy, M. (2015). Child Development Accounts and parental educational expectations for young children: Early evidence from a statewide social experiment. *Social Service Review, 89*(1), 99–137.

Lewis, M., O'Brien, M., Jones-Layman, A., O'Neill, E. A., & Elliott, W. (2017). Saving and educational asset building within a community-driven CSA Program: The case of Promise Indiana. *Poverty & Public Policy, 9*(2), 188–208.

Nam, Y., Kim, Y., Clancy, M., Zager, R., & Sherraden, M. (2013). Do Child Development Accounts promote account holding, saving, and asset accumulation for children's future? Evidence from a statewide randomized experiment. *Journal of Policy Analysis and Management, 32*(1), 6–33.

Sherraden, M. (1991). Assets and the poor: A new American welfare policy. Armonk, NY: M. E. Sharpe.

Sherraden, M. S. (2013). Building blocks of financial capability. In J. Birkenmaier, M. S. Sherraden, & J. Curley (Eds.), Financial education and capability: Research, education, policy, and practice (pp. 3–43). New York, NY: Oxford University Press.

Sherraden, M., Cheng, L.- C., Ssewamala, F. M., Kim, Y., Loke, V., Zou, L., Chowa., G., ... Han C.- K. (2018). International Child Development Accounts. *Encyclopedia of Social Work.* DOI:10.1093/acrefore/9780199975839.013.1261

Sherraden, M., Clancy, M., & Beverly, S. (2018). Taking Child Development Accounts to scale: Ten key policy design elements. St. Louis, MO: Center for Social Development, Washington University in St. Louis.

Index

Note: Page numbers in *italics* indicate a figure and page numbers in **bold** indicate a table on the corresponding page.